A CANCER
IN THE FAMILY

A CANCER IN THE FAMILY

Take Control of
Your Genetic Inheritance

THEODORA ROSS, M.D., PH.D.

AVERY
an imprint of Penguin Random House
New York

AVERY

an imprint of Penguin Random House LLC
375 Hudson Street
New York, New York 10014

First trade paperback edition, January 2017

Illustration credit: page 21, Darryl Leja, National Genome Research Institute

Most Avery books are available at special quantity discounts for bulk purchase for sales promotions, premiums, fund-raising, and educational needs. Special books or book excerpts also can be created to fit specific needs. For details, write SpecialMarkets@penguinrandomhouse.com.

Library of Congress Cataloging-in-Publication Data

Names: Ross, Theodora, author.
Title: A cancer in the family : take control of your genetic inheritance /
Theodora Ross.
Description: New York : Avery, an imprint of Penguin Random House, [2016]
Identifiers: LCCN 2015026294 | ISBN 9781101982839 (hardback)
Subjects: LCSH: Ross, Theodora—Health. | Cancer—Genetic aspects. |
Families—History. | Oncologists—United States—Biography. | BISAC:
HEALTH & FITNESS / Diseases / Cancer. | HEALTH & FITNESS / Diseases /
Genetic. | BIOGRAPHY & AUTOBIOGRAPHY / Personal Memoirs.
Classification: LCC RC268.4 .R68 2016 | DDC 616.99/4042—dc23
LC record available at http://lccn.loc.gov/2015026294

ISBN 9780147516909 (paperback)

Printed in the United States of America
1 3 5 7 9 10 8 6 4 2

BOOK DESIGN BY TANYA MAIBORODA

To my family.

I owe a huge debt of gratitude for the inspiration
provided by Grammy, Grumpy, Uncle Jack, and Bea.
I know that my use of their stories to help others
understand their own family's story and live longer,
healthier lives would have made them happy.
And to Sean, the family member
who read the chapters with critical care and
endorsed them with "Other than *Sports Illustrated*,
this is the only literature that made me cry."

AUTHOR'S NOTE: To protect the patients' privacy, I have changed the names of most patients and their families. I have also changed identifying details when necessary.

CONTENTS

FOREWORD

by SIDDHARTHA MUKHERJEE, M.D., PH.D.,
author of *The Emperor of All Maladies*

THEODORA ROSS'S EXTRAORDINARY BOOK on cancer genetics is an important contribution to the field. Allow me to introduce it with some historical background. Since the late 1970s, researchers have identified several genes that are implicated in cancer. In virtually all these cases, mutations in genes contribute to the abnormal physiology of growth that ultimately unleashes the cancerous transformation of a normal cell. Many of these mutations are acquired during our lifetimes—but, notably, some of these mutations are inherited in families.

The identification of heritable cancer-causing mutations has raised several quandaries that particularly haunt men and women with family histories of cancer. How many of these genes do we know—and how many remain unknown? What is the precise nature of risk associated with any one such gene? What tests or strategies can we deploy to reduce that risk? What if we carry a known cancer risk in our families, and yet do not know the gene involved in carrying the risk? And will we be able to test for such genes in ourselves or our children in the future?

Ross is especially qualified as a guide to these questions because of her extensive experience in the area as a physician, scientist, and cancer researcher. She completed her medical degree and a Ph.D. in biochemistry at Washington University. She trained in internal medicine at one of the preeminent hospitals at Harvard Medical School (the Brigham and Women's Hospital) and then in oncology at the Dana-Farber Cancer Institute, before launching her career in cancer genetics with the renowned leukemia researcher Gary Gilliland. In Gilliland's lab, she cloned a novel cancer gene that causes leukemia. Since 1999, she has been running her own independent laboratory, trying to understand the mechanisms by which cancer genes promote the transformation of normal cells into cancer cells. She was a professor at the University of Michigan and now leads the Cancer Genetics program at UT Southwestern in Dallas.

One of Ross's key successes has involved integrating the study of cancer genes in the laboratory to the care of cancer patients in the clinic. One such project involves identifying patients who are known to have a genetic predisposition to cancer but who do not have any known mutations in genes. By sequencing thousands of genes from such patients, Ross's team has identified a series of novel risk-increasing mutations. Her lab and the genetics program in Texas have established and published the first collection of sequences from 278 such patients, resulting in a treasure trove of genetic information.

But there's a deeper and more personal reason that makes this book particularly poignant and urgent: Ross has a BRCA1 mutation herself, and a strong family history of cancer. She has been living with knowledge of that mutation for twelve years, and traveling through the complicated landscape of anxieties, losses, avoidance, judgment calls, and empowering choices that come with a family history of cancer. This book is like having a comforting chat with a passionate doctor and researcher who is also your friend—the kind of friend who can weave together accessible science, personal stories, and practical suggestions.

Ross guides us through this landscape with astonishing personal honesty, clear thinking, openness, and persistence. She explains—with an empathy that can only arise from inhabiting the worlds of doctor and patient simultaneously—how all of us (professionals and laypeople alike), with or without a family history of cancer, need help understanding genetics. We need help digging up our family histories, confronting those histories, and making the decisions that will protect us and our families. By the time you finish this book, you will know about cancer genetics and how that knowledge can save your life.

Now that you have started this book, congratulations—you've also begun your own journey. Confronting a family history of cancer and thinking about the nuts and bolts of genetics can feel overwhelming. Ultimately, though, the knowledge you'll gain from this book is empowering. It can save your life, and the lives of the people you love most.

A CANCER
IN THE FAMILY

Chapter One

Knowledge That Can Save Your Life

SEVERAL YEARS AGO, when I was a researcher studying cancer cells and a doctor treating cancer patients, I had an experience that changed my life. That experience convinced me that people need more resources to help them understand inherited cancers and to help them assemble a plan of action when cancer appears to run in the family. This book is a result of the experience I'm about to describe, and it is here for you to use.

It was March 2004 and I was sitting with my husband, Sean, at the round table in my sixth-floor office at the University of Michigan's cancer center. I had a nicely sized office, with a desk decorated with a couple of computers and photos of lab members and special patients, as well as pictures of our family mugging for posterity. There were shelves that held trinkets from patients, along with yards of books about cancer biology and cancer care. When the phone on the table rang, Sean and I jumped. We knew that the incoming call would tell us the results of my own genetic test—that we would learn whether I was at risk for inherited cancer. I put the call on speakerphone so that both of us could hear the news. Neither one of us could sit still, so, without saying anything, we both stood up, walked to the window, and looked out at the snow.

I thought about what had brought me to that moment. Sean and I had been at the beach the previous summer when he pointed to a small spot on my leg. It had been there for a while, but Sean observed that it had changed in its appearance. After I got home, I decided to show it to a dermatologist, who said that he didn't know what it was but that he would remove it—not because he suspected cancer, but because that's what dermatologists do when there's something on your skin they don't recognize. A week later, I had a diagnosis: melanoma. Melanoma. *Me.* I've got the complexion of an Italian-Russian-Jewish mutt. My hair and eyes are dark brown and my skin tans deeply and easily. People with complexions like mine aren't supposed to get melanoma. Even the dermatologist was surprised. Without classic risk factors like pale skin and a history of sunburn, melanoma was very unlikely . . . unless an unseen genetic mutation had increased my risk. The melanoma was, fortunately, in an early stage and curable by surgery. But Sean urged me to consult with genetics experts.

I booked an appointment at a genetics clinic, telling myself I was just humoring Sean. Deep down, though, I knew that I should have had genetic testing years earlier. When I was in elementary school, I was stunned when my uncle Jack died of what my immediate family believed to be adrenal cancer. As I grew up, cancer made further appearances in my family, and I eventually realized that I wanted to become either a scientist who studied medical mysteries or a doctor who treated patients. Eventually, I went all the way and did both. I enrolled in the medical scientist M.D., Ph.D. training program at Washington University School of Medicine in St. Louis, which teaches students how to treat disease as well as how to research its causes and cures. By the time I graduated, I needed both hands to count the family members who'd developed cancer: not just Uncle Jack but also my mother, father, aunt, sister, and one of my brothers had come down with cancer of different kinds. When my beloved older sister, Bea, died of breast cancer at age thirty-eight, while I was still in medical training, I doubled down on my resolve.

In the years after Bea's death, I couldn't shake loose a series of questions: Was Bea's cancer sporadic, the kind of cancer that develops as a result of gene mutations, or changes, that arise by chance as we age? The vast majority of cancer cases—about 90 percent of them—are, in fact, sporadic. Or was it hereditary, meaning that one of our parents had passed down to Bea a genetic mutation that predisposed her to cancer? Because she was so young, the chances that it was hereditary were increased. If Bea's cancer was hereditary, I could have inherited the same mutation. The same went for my brothers and for Bea's children. And our cousins and their children. Cancer had already touched so many of us. Was my entire family at risk?

At the time Bea died, in the early 1990s, it was known that cancer syndromes could be passed down through families, but the technology for testing DNA to spot a mutation didn't exist. I spent a lot of time debating with myself, first mounting the argument that the various cancers in our family were caused by a mutation—and then deciding that those cancers didn't fit any of the patterns that tend to appear when a mutation is present in a family. We'd just been unlucky. It happens.

By the time I found myself sitting in my office with Sean, Bea's death was behind us by more than a decade, and I'd become both an oncologist and a cancer biologist. I was hungry to study the "breast cancer genes," BRCA1 and BRCA2. These genes are mutated in 1 percent of the wider population, but certain subsets of the population are more likely to have these mutations, such as people of

Ashkenazi Jewish descent. People who carry mutant forms of either of these genes have a very high risk of developing breast and ovarian cancer; they also have a modestly increased risk for a variety of other cancers. But the studies I wanted to do required funding I didn't have—and unrestricted access to carefully collected clinical material. Both privacy laws and medical ethics made that access limited and difficult to get. So up until that snowy March day in 2004, I had adjusted my professional goal. I was busily focused on the basic mechanisms that cause normal cells to transform into cancer cells and what makes some cancer cells resistant to targeted drugs. I cared for breast cancer patients at all stages of the disease. It wasn't the work I had initially set out to do, but it was challenging, educational, and useful. I felt safe there, in my warm cocoon of an office. Safe and busy. Too busy to keep thinking about whether my family carried a mutation that causes hereditary cancer. I had too much on my mind to bother with genetic counseling. I was too distracted, now that genetic testing had become available, to submit a sample of my DNA to a lab.

At least, I was distracted until my melanoma diagnosis. And that's how Sean and I ended up there, in my office, waiting to find out if I carried a mutation for cancer, to find out if I might be at risk for the same kinds of cancers that had plagued my family.

"Hello?" The voice of Heather, my genetic counselor, came through the line. Heather is soft-spoken but, thankfully, she is also direct. (There's nothing worse than a genetic counselor who can't deliver tough news.) "I'm so sorry to tell you this, but given that your test results were returned so quickly, you've probably already figured out that you have a mutation."

In fact, I hadn't figured that out. I'd been savoring the final days of denial.

"Unfortunately," she said, "it's the BRCA1 5382insC Ashkenazi mutation." In the world of cancer genetics, this is one of the most common BRCA mutations, particularly prevalent among people of Ashkenazi descent. Inherited mutations that predispose people to cancer can occur in many different genes; each gene and each mutation produces its own set of risks for different kinds of cancers. Several types of mutations can occur in the BRCA1 gene alone. You may have heard of them; they have unpoetic names that tend to make the eyes glaze over: BRCA1 185delAG and BRCA1 1556del and BRCA2 4449del and so on.

Some inherited cancer mutations increase your risk by a moderate amount, and not every mutation is cause for immediate action. Some are best managed through screening and watchful waiting. But the BRCA1 5382insC (pronounced if spelled out: *be-are-see-ay-one, fifty-three eighty-two insertion see*) mutation increases your chances for breast and ovarian cancers by a large factor. For example, the average woman has a 1 to 2 percent risk of developing ovarian cancer over a lifetime; for a woman with the BRCA1 5382insC mutation, that risk leaps up to 40 percent. And whereas the average woman has a 12 percent risk of developing breast cancer over her lifetime, someone with a BRCA1 mutation has a risk somewhere between 50 and 87 percent, depending on her family history. BRCA1 5382insC increases the risk of other cancers, too—like melanoma and prostate cancer.

Ironically, the mutation's nastiness was one reason I'd longed to study BRCA1, which is the normal, nonmutated version of the gene, the one most people carry in their cells. As with many things, the importance of BRCA1 to the normal life of the cell isn't easily appreciated until it's gone—or mutated. A normal BRCA1 gene helps protect us from cancer by working to keep our genetic material intact. When BRCA1 is mutated, its function is impaired, and that protection against cancer disappears or declines. It's as if a door that has been locked is opened, and cancer is invited to walk in. Cancer might not take up the invitation, but there's a good chance it will. If we could understand more about how BRCA1 works under normal circumstances, it could lead to rational strategies for the prevention and treatment of cancers that tend to develop alongside BRCA1 mutations.

Sensing that I might have temporarily forgotten everything I knew about genetics, Heather ushered us through the logic. As she had suggested, the BRCA1 5382insC mutation is most common in people who are descended from Ashkenazi Jews, an ethnic subgroup of Jews who, until the last century, lived mostly in central and eastern Europe.

"It must have come from your dad," Heather said. "Your mom's not of Jewish descent, but he is. This mutation would explain plenty of the cancers on your dad's side of the family and your melanoma. Of course, your sister, Bea, must have had the mutation, too; that's why she developed breast cancer at such a young age. Theo, this means you have a high risk for ovarian and breast cancer. We suggest you consider a double mastectomy and removal of the ovaries to reduce your risk. I'll send you the papers with the data so you can see that evidence supports these recommendations. And you'll need to notify your brothers and other paternal relatives so that they and their children can be tested."

It was a moment that could have been inspired by the cheesy movies Bea and I had watched together as kids: *When the gene hunter becomes the hunted.* I'd been studying cancer all my adult life, and now it turned out that I was carrying a cancer mutation around inside my cells. At first, I was shocked, and then I felt a little exposed in front of Heather and Sean, and then I felt embarrassed for feeling exposed. The psychology of bad news suggests that the next emotion on deck would be anger or fear or grief, but what I felt was *release.*

And this was the experience that changed my life. After years of not knowing how to think about my risk of cancer, and years of trying to quiet the drumbeat of worry that banged around in the back of my mind, I knew. Instead of a vague anxiety, instead of spending mental energy on denial, I finally had clear, solid information. The feeling of purpose that had driven my career choice refreshed itself. I could feel a to-do list assembling itself in my head. There were medical appointments and decisions to make. I realized almost immediately that I would go for the double mastectomy and the removal of my ovaries. As an oncologist, I had cared for patients with aggressive, difficult-to-treat breast and ovarian cancers, and I'd watched my own sister die. I had also recommended these pro-phylactic surgeries (the removal of an organ that is prone to cancer) to patients in my situation; now I saw the surgeries as my own life-line, and I grabbed on tight. I knew that Bea's children, although they were still young, would have the opportunity to be tested when they were older. A negative result would give them peace of mind. A positive one would bring them options that their mother never had. I realized that, for the first time in my family's history, my family would have power against the diseases that have harmed us.

There was one more thing. I'd always wanted to study the BRCA1 gene and the mutations that disable it, but I couldn't—at least, not in the way I wanted to—because I wasn't ethically or legally able to ask another person to fork over his or her genetic material for my endless, unrestricted study. Now I didn't have to ask another person for genetic material. I could study myself. As it turned out, this moment—*when the hunter became the hunted*—was the moment when I became exactly who I'd always wanted to be.

I've written this book because it took me too long to arrive at that moment. Despite my background in the field, it wasn't until more than a decade after losing my sister that I understood what my family's history of cancer meant for us and for the generations to come. Now, as an oncologist, cancer gene hunter, cancer survivor, and the carrier of a cancer mutation, I want to help people like me and people like you. I don't want anyone to have to wait as long as I did. For years, I had been stuck in an unsettling, unhelpful state of not knowing. That's a shame, because knowing can help you manage your risk. You might have heard that there is nothing you can do to stop cancer from coming—but that's simply not true. The vast majority of people with inherited cancer syndromes can reduce their risk through a range of options that include surgeries, screenings, drug regimens, and lifestyle changes. In the most stunning instances, the risk of cancer can drop from nearly 100 percent to almost zero. It's incredibly common to avoid looking into a family history of cancer because of a fear of what you might find. I had thought that knowing would make me miserable, but it didn't. It energized me and made me effective. And it's not just me; I have seen the same positive effect over and over with my patients.

If cancer runs in your family, or if you think it might, this book will help you determine the steps you need to take. In the pages to come, you'll learn:

- What you need to know about inherited cancer, including the science of DNA and how cancer mutations are passed through families,
- How to spot the telltale patterns that signal cancer mutations,
- Why it's more important than ever to know your genetic inheritance,
- How to handle the family politics of cancer secrecy,
- The psychology of self-deception,
- The reasons medical professionals sometimes add to the haze of half-truths around family cancer histories, and
- How to use your genetic information to your best advantage.

Along the way I'll show you people, including my patients and my family members, who have found ways to unlock the information they need to make wise choices. There is no one-size-fits-all in the world of cancer genetics. It's OK for different people to make different choices. I hope to help you determine what is best for you.

As I'll explain, denial was a significant reason it took me so long to learn about my mutation. But it was not the only reason. I also lost valuable time because both professionals and laypeople tend to talk about inherited cancer using indirect, cautious language that I often misunderstood. I will be direct and open with you; I will be as straight with you as my counselor Heather was with me. The clear exchange of knowledge is the only way for any of us to have real power.

Why Not "Just Get Tested"?

At any given moment, thirteen million people in the United States have cancer. For each of those thirteen million, there are family members who are wondering: Is this cancer part of a pattern? Does cancer run in my family? Am I at risk?

If you are asking these questions, you are in the same shoes I stood in. If you are like me, you may be frustrated that the rest of the world believes you have a clear path ahead of you. Take a family medical history, talk to your doctor, get tested if necessary, get a definitive answer.

As you may have already discovered, it's not that easy. I spent years training in both science and medicine—with a specialty in cancer—and even I found that these steps are far more complicated than they seem. Cancer is a big, unwieldy topic; so is genetics. There's so much to get your head around and so many possible obstacles in your path.

Some of those obstacles are pretty close to home. For example, there's a general feeling that a person who's worried about a cancer mutation should "just get tested." It's a simple concept in theory, but the reality is more complicated. Although it's possible to get an over-the-counter genetic test on your own, the labs that perform these tests are forbidden by law from interpreting most of the results for you. The law is there to protect you against interpretations that are inaccurate or lead to actions that are harmful. An over-the-counter lab can tell you that you have a possible mutation in a particular gene, but you wouldn't know whether that gene variation is harmful or benign, or whether it's a variation whose significance is not yet known. (As I'll explain later in the book, the vast majority of rare genetic variations from what we consider "normal" are harmless, and there are many, many mutations we don't yet understand.) If you don't know what a genetic change *means*, you don't have a very helpful piece of information; you just have a bunch of numbers and letters on a page.

For that reason, it's far better to work through a doctor or a genetic counselor. But one of the most counterproductive things you can do is send your blood to a lab, or let your doctor send your blood to a lab, without first understanding what syndromes and mutations you're most likely at risk for. These labs analyze the genes that are most likely to be mutated, which varies from person to person; without accurate knowledge of your family history, you could easily end up getting the wrong test—and, possibly, a false sense of security. To determine what genes are most likely to have mutations, you (along with a genetic counselor) need to be able to spot the patterns common to familial cancers. Even if you already know that you have a mutation, it's important to get a family history. A family history helps predict the risk of a mutation in any particular individual. Without a family history, you may know that you have an increased risk, but you may not know whether your risk is on the high end, the low end, or somewhere in the middle. That information—where you fall in the range of increased risk—can affect the choices you make about how to protect yourself.

For these reasons, you need a family health history that is as thorough as possible. Taking a family history sounds like a neatly defined task. Until you run into family members who lie to you or who make it emotionally perilous to discuss health issues.

At first this concern can sound outdated. Cancer secrecy? Cancer shame? In the *twenty-first century*? It's been forty years since Betty Ford announced that she'd had a mastectomy. Two decades since the first cancer-awareness ribbon fluttered. More than a decade since Katie Couric's colonoscopy was broadcast live. And eight years since *Merriam-Webster* named "oversharing" its word of the year. It's been a long, long time since "cancer" was a word that made nice ladies blanch and gaze down at their shoes.

And yet. We do keep secrets about cancer, and it's incredibly common to run into other problems—vagueness, bad information, bad feelings, legal issues—that keep people from understanding their risk. In addition to now happily researching the normal and abnormal biology of BRCA and other cancer genes in the lab, I work with a team of counselors and high-risk cancer patients of all kinds. *Every day* we see patients who are blindsided by a diagnosis of inherited cancer. These are people who have already missed their chances for early detection and preventive treatment. Now they're scrambling to learn enough about their histories to determine if they are at risk for future cancers—and to write an accurate history for the next generation. Some examples: A young woman is surprised when she develops ovarian cancer, apparently out of the blue; she then learns that her aunt also had ovarian cancer in early adulthood but had been so embarrassed that she didn't tell anyone about it. A son gets colon cancer at twenty and finds out the man he's always thought was his father is not, in fact, his biological father, and that his bloodline father died of colon cancer—also at age twenty. Another family doesn't realize that they have a significant history of prostate cancers. That's because some branches of the family refuse to speak to other branches; no one has put together the full medical history.

In my own case, my family had no serious estrangements, and our worries about cancer actually pulled us closer together. Yet somehow we had unwittingly spread half-truths about our family history, carried secret histories about our ancestry, and ignored our best instincts when those instincts were inconvenient. (I was especially guilty of that last charge.) We weren't the only ones to participate in the concealment of our inheritance. Along the way, doctors and researchers helped us keep the truth from ourselves. There was no conspiracy here—just a human tendency to avoid pain and awkward discussions. When you're looking for patterns that suggest inherited mutations, this kind of misinformation can send you miles down the wrong path. Difficulty figuring out the family history is the rule, not the exception.

What about getting cancer information from the Internet? What sounds like a good plan is actually an exercise in frustration. You can't Google your way to an understanding of family cancer. The few sites and pages that specifically address family cancer don't tell you what you really need to know. "Get counseling," they chirp. "Get tested!" But they don't offer thorough information about the nature of hereditary cancers and the kinds of patterns that can alert you to the possibility that a cancer syndrome is being passed down through the generations of your family.

For example, there's a lot of chatter online and in doctors' offices about mutations in BRCA1 and BRCA2, the breast cancer genes. But there are other mutations that can lead to breast cancer—and BRCA mutations can lead to more than just breast cancer. Also, they can affect both men and women. So if your father has had prostate cancer and your uncle has been diagnosed with melanoma, you may carry a BRCA mutation—even if you're a man. Both men and women with BRCA mutations are at risk for a variety of cancers, and so are adult children who inherit a broken BRCA gene from their parent. But most websites and other public sources of information offer a more limited view. In the pages to come, you'll get the details you need to investigate your family's patterns and understand what you find.

Not knowing about a genetic predisposition to cancer, or not understanding the significance of that predisposition, *matters*. It matters because there is so much good to be discovered in that knowledge. As I found, learning your genetic inheritance may feel daunting, but in the end it can give you a sense of release, an ability to go out into the world with less fear and more confidence. It grants you the power to make lifesaving decisions, both for yourself and for the generations to come.

A Family History of Cancer
Is a Powerful Tool for Better Health

It takes courage to look at a family history of cancer. A major reason people fail to assess their genetic inheritance is that it's hard for them to see the upside—to imagine that life can be better, not worse, if they discover they're at increased risk for cancer.

But a family history of cancer can be fashioned into one of the best health tools available in contemporary medicine. It's right up there with clean water, sanitary sewers, and childhood immunizations in terms of its ability to profoundly improve your health. For example, my mutation predicts a 50 to 87 percent risk of developing breast cancer over a lifetime. Because of my family cancer history, I was probably on the high end of that range. Prophylactic surgeries and screening have cut down my risk for breast cancer so that it's now the same as that of someone in the normal population, which is about 12 percent over a lifetime. Possibly my risk is even lower.

When I tell people that I work with patients at a high risk for familial cancer, they pull a somber face and murmur that the work must be tough. Sometimes it is. But if you could see what goes on in our cancer genetics clinics at the University of Texas Southwestern Medical Center's Comprehensive Cancer Center, you'd discover that, for most people, genetic knowledge is a source of relief and hope and *action*. Here are some of the scenes that unfold in our clinics:

- A forty-year-old woman with Lynch syndrome (she carries a mutation that predisposes her to colon and other cancers) walks into the clinic, weeping. She is afraid that she will get colon cancer, die early, and leave her young son motherless. We explain that a yearly colonoscopy will remove any precancerous polyps and almost certainly let her enjoy a relatively normal life span. Her face softens with relief.

- Tricia, a single mother, has brought her two sons in for testing after a long delay. Tricia has Li-Fraumeni syndrome (she carries a TP53 [tumor protein p53] mutation that can lead to a variety of cancers), and she dreads the thought that her sons might have the same. She learns that her younger son is in the clear. The other is not. But a series of annual tests will help doctors monitor his health and intervene early if a problem arises. Tricia's free-floating worry is replaced by relief for her younger son and a plan that will help her protect her older one.

- A young man in his twenties, whose family is studded with the kinds of cancer horror stories that make all of us blink back tears, meets with a genetic counselor. From previous genetic testing, we know that the cause is a hereditary syndrome called familial adenomatous polyposis. Most of the family members have received this news with denial, and we can guess why: Regular, frequent colonoscopies are not enough to protect a person with this particular syndrome.

The entire colon must be removed. But today, the young man is here to be tested, and he's prepared to take action if he has the mutation. No matter what the result, this clinic visit will allow him to refocus on his teaching career, marry his long-time girlfriend, and help the rest of his family face their risk.

- Janice, a thirty-nine-year-old law professor with HER2-positive breast cancer, has just learned she has a BRCA1 mutation. Although her tumor is not a type commonly associated with BRCA mutations and she has no family history of cancer, we test her because of her young age. To the surprise of both of us, she is positive for a BRCA1 mutation. At first a fountain of spontaneous tears blurs the BRCA1-positive report. "How could this be?" she asks, staring at the page. After our discussion of what it all means, she transforms from shocked to enthralled. The BRCA1 mutation guides treatment of her tumor, and awareness of it can prevent future cancers for her, her children, and her other family members. We adjust her chemotherapy to include cisplatin, a drug not routinely used for breast cancer *except* in the presence of BRCA mutations. Because tumors with BRCA mutations don't fully repair DNA, cisplatin exploits this defect to destroy the tumor cells without killing normal cells. Newer drugs, such as PARP (poly ADP ribose polymerase) inhibitors, target a similar weakness in the cancer cells. I'll describe these newer drugs in detail in chapter 7, when I discuss how patients, their families, and their doctors can work together to find new avenues for cancer prevention and cancer treatment.

Knowing *is* better than not knowing. Clarity is better than confusion. There are options for cancer prevention and risk management that give you much more control over your health. Because having an inherited mutation can mean choosing how to manage your risk, this book will describe decision-making strategies that can help you make sound choices and go forward with confidence. We'll also take a look at the way cancer treatments increasingly depend on an intimate knowledge of *you*, and take a look at both the hype and the realistic hopes for treatments specific to your genetic inheritance.

Finally, the book will explore the promise and perils of today's cancer research and argue that those of us with inherited cancer mutations have an obligation to share our data—not just with our families but also with the physicians and researchers who may be our best hope for an eventual cure. After all, in a genetic sense, we are all part of the same family tree. When we withhold our information, we withhold it from everyone who is hoping for better cancer prevention and treatment options.

Millions of people see cancer in their family members and wonder, "Am I next? Are my children?" It can be hard to know what to do with these worries. I hope to give you positive, practical help, because finding the answers can give you the ability to shape your destiny.

Chapter Two

The Double Helix:
Biology Isn't Destiny

IN ANCIENT GREECE, Hippocrates speculated that cancer was caused by a bodily substance he called "black bile." Black bile could supposedly be generated by certain foods and activities. In the 1800s, physicians talked about how tumors were caused by "cancer juice." Later, doctors believed that cancer began with a physical injury to the affected body part. Over the years, theories about the causes of cancer have been promoted, discarded, and dug up again. In the 1980s and '90s, one particular notion clicked with the reading public: Cancer is caused by toxic stress, particularly resentment. Bernie Siegel's book *Love, Medicine, and Miracles* was a driver of the idea that unresolved past emotional traumas can build up, and build up some more, and gather a kind of mass—and eventually they express themselves in a solid physical form, as a cancerous tumor.

My mother, now called Grammy by all in the family, saw stress as an explanation for why my sister, Bea, had developed breast cancer at the young age of thirty-five. Actually, I think Grammy took

Freud's famous notion that "biology is destiny"—he meant that women's bodies inevitably tie them to pregnancy, child rearing, and homemaking—and put her own special spin on it. She believed that when talented women allow themselves to follow conventional lives of raising children and caregiving, they experience extreme stress. She blamed this stress for Bea's breast cancer. Grammy would have found backup in the 1984 best-selling book *You Can Heal Your Life,* by Louise Hay, which echoed Grammy's thinking and tied it together with Bernie Siegel's: "The breasts represent the mothering principle. When there are problems with the breasts, it usually means we are 'over-mothering' either a person, a place, a thing, or an experience. . . . If cancer is involved, then there is also deep resentment." I'll bring up the stress issue again later, but right here I want to state clearly that stress doesn't cause cancer. Even though Siegel and Hay offered their theories with a compassionate spirit, they misled their readers. Neither author explained that their ideas, in fact, were just as unsupported by science and just as superficial as Freud's "biology is destiny" proclamation.

It's possible that stress can slightly increase your risk for cancer. However, the biology tells us that this is a much smaller risk factor than variables like cancer mutations, smoking, obesity, or alcohol consumption. When people believe that stress causes cancer—and this belief is still around—they are often distracted from the real steps they can take to understand and manage cancer risks. Another problem is that people with cancer can begin to feel guilty, believing that they've brought cancer on themselves by being unable to manage their stress.

At about the same time that there was a national kitchen-table conversation about cancer and stress, I was a student in the medical-scientist training program at Washington University School of Medicine in St. Louis and learning a completely different approach to cancer, one that would become more detailed over the years as medical scientists learned more about the biology of cancer and, especially, how it can be handed down through families. As I was studying medicine, I didn't realize that cancer was about to become even more personal for me—that it would touch, and deeply wound, my family again and again.

I'm sharing this part of my family's story to illustrate the things that everyone with a family history of cancer needs to know: the science of DNA and inherited mutations, the signs that inherited mutations may be causing family cancer, and the kinds of syndromes that can result from an inherited mutation. Even more, it's crucial to be as clear and honest about these things as you can, starting at home with family conversations and moving into doctor's offices, online medical sites, and research labs. When it comes to cancer—and especially to family cancer—you've got to be clearheaded about the information that's founded on good science and the ideas that are just guesses.

Every Cancer Is Genetic

What I learned in school also linked cancer, biology, and destiny, but in a completely different way than my mother's ideas did. "Cancer" is an umbrella term for hundreds of different disorders, but what all cancers have in common is runaway cell growth. Many cells are supposed to be able to divide and reproduce; that's how we grow new tissues to repair ones that have been damaged or to replace old cells that have worn out. Cells in regenerating tissues (like the skin and blood) are supposed to live out their natural life span and then die, with new cells replacing them. But something can warp a cell's mission and tell the cell to keep dividing. Instead of doing their part to help your body stay healthy, these cells proliferate out of control, forming tumors rather than just replacing the cells that normally turn over in your tissues. In metastasis, cancer cells develop the abnormal ability to migrate throughout the body, implanting, proliferating, and disrupting other tissues.

What causes cells to change from healthy and normal to cancerous? It begins in the genes. Sometimes you'll hear people say casually that "so-and-so's cancer is genetic," but that's misleading. *Every* cancer is genetic. Every cancer involves mutations in genes.

A Short (Very Short) Tutorial in Genetics

If you think of cancer as something that is too complicated to understand, you will only increase your worries and fear. It's true that cancer is extraordinarily complex, but it's not hard to get a handle on the basics of DNA and cancer biology. Genes are segments of deoxyribonucleic acid, or DNA. Think of DNA as two long strips that twist around each other, forming the classic double-helix shape that you may have learned about in school. Now imagine that each of these strips is made up of four different letters that are each repeated thousands of times. Those four letters, which each represent a different molecule or nucleotide, are A, T, C, and G. The precise order of these nucleotides determines what amino acids make up our proteins, and differences in the composition of our proteins are what cause variations in traits like eye color, height, and cancer predisposition. BRCA1 mutations alter the amino acid composition of the BRCA1 protein, impairing its function and its ability to repair DNA damage in cells.

Genes are like sections in a cell's instructional manual. They determine the structure of proteins, which regulate all aspects of cellular function, such as cell division and cell survival. They also determine the type of job the cell performs. For example, a liver cell metabolizes toxins, a stomach cell secretes acid, and a brain cell helps you think. Only a subset of genes is turned on in each cell. The reason blood cells are different from skin cells is that different genes

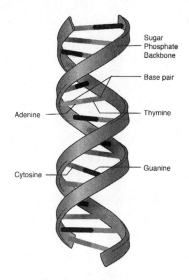

Sugar Phosphate Backbone

Base pair

Adenine

Thymine

Cytosine

Guanine

are turned on in each cell type, making different proteins. For example, the gene for the protein hemoglobin is turned on in red blood cells but not in other cells, rendering red blood cells uniquely red in color and able to transport oxygen throughout the body. Every person's DNA—and the combinations of genes that make up their DNA—is unique. It's the code that gives me my dark brown eyes and hair, and it might even contribute to my sense of humor, which is not so dark.

You have two copies of most of your genes, one copy from each of your parents.

But the letters of one or both copies can get mixed up and written in the wrong way. These mix-ups are mutations. As a cell divides and reproduces itself, it passes the mutation on to the next cell, which then reproduces itself, and so on and so on. The word "mutations" conjures up images of two-headed monsters that eat Tokyo, but they're actually very common. We all have them. In fact, we all have *lots* of them. The vast majority of mutations don't cause cancer.

Most don't have any effect on your body at all. But some can lead to cancer. The mutations that are most closely associated with an increased cancer risk are the ones that affect cell growth, cell survival, or the ability to repair damaged DNA. Before cancer can begin, a cell usually needs to accumulate several mutations like these. Conventional wisdom among physicians is that a cell needs multiple mutations of a particular kind—the kind that alters the functions of genes that regulate the cell's survival and proliferation—before it becomes cancerous. That's because when you boil it right down, the most basic differences between cancer cells and normal cells are that cancer cells proliferate when they shouldn't and survive when they shouldn't.

What causes the mutations that can lead to cancer? Some factors are clear. Certain types of ionizing radiation, like X-rays and ultraviolet rays, can mutate DNA. Some chemicals, like the ones found in cigarettes and asbestos, also cause mutations. Alcohol intake is linked to increased cancer incidence, though the way it promotes cancer isn't yet clear. Not every mutation leads to cancer. Most mutations don't have any effect at all. That's why infrequent X-rays are very unlikely to cause cancer.

Inherited vs. Sporadic Cancer

Every day, your body experiences twenty million cell divisions. Most of the time, the division process works smoothly. But every now and then, the cells make mistakes as they copy their DNA to pass on to their daughter cells. The strands of DNA pair up in the wrong way. Letters are added or dropped. A piece breaks off and gets reinserted at the wrong point. Copying errors like these cause mutations, along with errors when chromosomes pair up during cell division. External factors (like ionizing radiation and certain chemicals as mentioned above) are significant causes of mutations, too, because they cause direct breaks in the DNA that increase copying errors. No matter how a mutation happens, when a cell with an unrepaired mutation divides, it passes that mutation to its offspring cells, and those cells pass the mutation along to *their* offspring. In this way, mutations can accumulate over time. Moreover, mutations that impede DNA repair increase the probability of subsequent mutations, and mutations that increase cellular proliferation or survival allow the mutant cells to outcompete normal cells. Accumulate enough mutations of a certain kind, and cancer develops.

Most cancers are sporadic, arising as a result of mutations that accumulate in cells as a consequence of exposure to environmental mutagens (agents in your environment that can mutate your DNA, like cigarette smoke or ultraviolet light from the sun) or random bad luck (some mutations occur by chance when cells replicate their DNA during cell division). Sporadic cancers are distinct from inherited cancers that arise in large part as a result of mutations that are passed to you from your parents. Inherited cancers (defined as cancers in patients with a known cancer-predisposing gene mutation) make up about 10 percent of cancer cases. You can be born with a particular kind of genetic mutation that is passed down from parent to child, like a BRCA mutation. Instead of being acquired by one cell in one tissue and then passed on to its offspring cells, an inherited mutation exists in almost every cell of your body from the minute you are conceived. People with inherited cancer-causing mutations are born with an increased risk of cancer because their cells have a head start in the mutation department. (It's possible that some sporadic mutations can be handed from parent to child. Data show that smoking—even secondhand smoking—can cause cancer mutations in germ cells such as sperm. These mutations can therefore be passed down to subsequent generations. In case I haven't made this point clear yet, it's a bad idea to smoke.)

There are hundreds of known inherited genes that, when

mutated, make you more susceptible to cancers of different types. But Freud had it wrong, at least when it comes to cancer: Biology is not the same as destiny. Having an inherited mutation does not mean that you will definitely get cancer. Whether or not you get cancer depends on a mixture of variables, some of which you control (such as whether or not you smoke) and some of which you don't (such as what other kinds of mutations you inherit or acquire by chance). How often do your cells make replication errors when dividing, and what kinds of errors do they make? Are you exposed to carcinogens that could cause mutations that can push your cells further toward cancer? For example, Rosalind Franklin, a scientist who helped discover the structure of DNA in the 1950s, died from ovarian cancer when she was only thirty-seven years old. Sometimes people argue over whether her cancer was caused by an inherited mutation or by repeated exposure to X-rays, which she used to take photographs of DNA. (At the time it was not understood that ionizing radiation causes DNA damage and that repeated exposure can lead to cancer, so scientists working with X-rays didn't use protective equipment.) Genetic testing wasn't available during Franklin's life, so we can only speculate, but there's a good chance that her cancer was caused by both factors. Cancer that appears at a young age can be a sign of an inherited mutation—plus, Franklin was of Ashkenazi Jewish descent, and this population has a much higher incidence of BRCA mutations. A BRCA mutation could have given her cancer a head start, and exposure to X-rays could have sped her cells toward a cancerous state.

In addition to environmental exposures, your family history of cancer, *even* if you have a known mutation, is important. A strong family history of cancer suggests that you may have more than one cancer-predisposing mutation, which compounds the chance that cancer will develop. We need further research to understand why some people with BRCA mutations or other cancer-predisposing mutations are more prone to cancer than others who carry the same mutation in their DNA.

Sometimes when cancer appears to run in families, there's no inherited mutation at all. There's another explanation, like sharing risk factors. Several of the family members may have been exposed to radon or asbestos or cigarette smoke. Sometimes it's just bad luck. Cancer is a common illness, and many people acquire cancer mutations over the course of their lives. Sometimes this happens to several people in one family, for no particular reason that we can identify, especially if people live long enough to accumulate the necessary series of acquired mutations.

But when there's an inherited mutation that puts many family members at a higher risk of particular types of cancers, it still doesn't mean that everyone in the family will have the inherited mutation or get cancer. Everyone gets two copies of genes, one from each parent. When you have a child, you pass down just one of those copies to the child—and the other parent contributes the second copy. So, if you have an inherited mutation, your child has a fifty-fifty chance of getting that mutation from you. Furthermore, a person can have a cancer-predisposing mutation and never get cancer but still pass the predisposition on to his or her children. It may look like the mutation can jump generations, but it doesn't. You can inherit a cancer mutation even from a parent who's never had cancer.

Does Cancer Run in Your Family? Look for These Signs

Patterns tend to emerge in families with inherited mutations—outward signs that suggest the family is genetically susceptible to particular kinds of cancers. Here are some clues that suggest an inherited cancer gene is traveling in a family:

- Cancer has appeared in your family members at an unusually young age (say, colon cancer or breast cancer before age fifty).
- Several blood relatives have the same type of cancer.
- A person in your family has experienced more than one kind of cancer.
- Cancer has independently appeared in both of a set of paired organs (both breasts or both kidneys, for example).
- Several people in your family have had an unusual or rare kind of cancer.
- People in your family have had specific birth defects, including certain skin growths and bone disorders that are associated with inherited cancer mutations.
- One or both sides of your family are of Ashkenazi Jewish descent, as this ethnic group has an increased chance of carrying a mutant cancer gene.

The more of these clues that have appeared in your family, and the more often they appear on the same side of your family tree, the higher the possibility that an inherited defective cancer gene is at work.

As you look over this list, keep in mind that cancer in a distant relative is less concerning than cancer in a closer one, because you're more likely to inherit genes from people who sit nearer to you on the family tree. Also, look at whether patterns emerge from people on the same side of the family, because you're looking for genes that are getting passed down through blood relatives. Breast cancer that appears in two aunts on your mother's side is a stronger cause for concern than breast cancer that appears in one aunt on your mother's side and one on your father's.

It might seem logical that a mutation in a specific gene would always lead to the same type of cancer, but that's rarely how it works. The mutations we're talking about don't directly cause a single type of cancer. They instead create conditions that increase the likelihood that cancer will develop, and the type of cancer that develops can vary not only with the type of gene but also from person to person. There are about fifty inherited cancer syndromes. Here, I've listed some of the most common, along with the name of the mutated gene or genes and the main cancers that tend to appear. Remember, a doctor isn't going to order tests for *all* the cancer syndromes on this list. First, you, your genetic counselor, and your doctor have to narrow things down to the most likely possibilities. That begins with information you supply about your family's cancer history.

Take a look to see if your family has cancers that fall into any of these patterns. As I'll explain in the chapters to come, genetic counselors are trained to help you with this process of identifying patterns.

Inherited Cancer Syndromes (adapted from the National Cancer Institute)

Hereditary breast cancer and ovarian cancer syndrome
ASSOCIATED GENES: BRCA1 and BRCA2
ASSOCIATED CANCERS: breast, ovarian, prostate, and pancreatic cancers, as well as melanoma

Familial malignant melanoma syndrome
ASSOCIATED GENES: CDKN2A and CDK4
ASSOCIATED CANCERS: melanoma, brain, and pancreatic cancer

Li-Fraumeni syndrome
ASSOCIATED GENE: TP53
ASSOCIATED CANCERS: breast cancer, soft-tissue sarcoma, osteosarcoma (bone cancer), leukemia, brain tumors,

adrenocortical carcinoma (cancer of the adrenal glands), and other cancers

Cowden syndrome (PTEN hamartoma tumor syndrome)
ASSOCIATED GENE: PTEN
ASSOCIATED CANCERS: breast, thyroid, endometrial, and other cancers

Lynch syndrome (hereditary nonpolyposis colorectal cancer syndrome)
ASSOCIATED GENES: MLH1, MSH2, MSH6, PMS2, and EPCAM
ASSOCIATED CANCERS: colorectal, endometrial, ovarian, small intestine, stomach, and bladder cancers

Familial adenomatous polyposis
ASSOCIATED GENE: APC
ASSOCIATED CANCERS: colorectal cancer and multiple nonmalignant colon polyps

Multiple endocrine neoplasia type 1 (MEN1)
ASSOCIATED GENE: MEN1
ASSOCIATED CANCERS: pancreatic neuroendocrine, parathyroid and pituitary gland tumors

Multiple endocrine neoplasia type 2 (MEN2)
ASSOCIATED GENE: RET
ASSOCIATED CANCERS: medullary thyroid cancer and pheochromocytoma (adrenal gland tumor)

Von Hippel–Lindau syndrome
ASSOCIATED GENE: VHL

ASSOCIATED CANCERS: kidney cancers, neuroendocrine tumors, hemangioblastomas, and pheochromocytomas

I've included a longer list, with more detailed information about the patterns and specific family clues that are associated with each syndrome, at the back of this book. As you begin to track down your family history, I urge you to take a look at these, especially the ones that seem to apply to your situation. For now, though, what's important is to have a bird's-eye view of hereditary cancer syndromes and to understand that the patterns of cancer in your family can be important clues about your own genetic inheritance.

Cancer and Family Secrets

In 1993, when I graduated from the M.D., Ph.D. training program and was psyching myself up for my internship and residency, researchers were just beginning to prove that cancers like the ones in my family could be handed down through mutations in specific genes. In the 1960s, both Lynch syndrome, which increases the risk of colon cancer, and Li-Fraumeni syndrome, an extremely rare disorder that greatly increases the chances of breast cancer, sarcoma (a rare kind of cancer of connective tissue), leukemia, and cancer of the adrenal glands, were identified as having a familial basis. And then in the 1990s scientists began pinpointing some of the actual genes at work and identifying other cancer syndromes.

By the spring of 1993, one of my brothers, Alex, and my sister, Bea, had been diagnosed with cancer, and for a while it looked as if both of them had recovered. At age thirty, Alex developed metastatic testicular cancer; he was treated with platinum-based chemotherapy, dealt with its side effects, and survived. Bea, who was originally diagnosed with breast cancer two years after Alex's diagnosis, had also endured chemotherapy and gone into remission.

Alex was engaged to be married, and Bea had been busy growing her family, working as a computer scientist, and volunteering for a cancer foundation. I was in a long-term relationship, wondering about marriage and children, and thinking about how to shape my career path. I knew that I wanted to study cancer, but in medical research, a single-minded, narrow focus is highly prized, and I wasn't sure where I wanted to aim that focus.

All the while, the cancers in my family were at the back of my mind. As I packed up my things and drove from St. Louis to my residency in Boston, I obsessively built up and then broke down the case that our family had an inherited predisposition to cancer. This was a mostly intellectual exercise for me, because even if there was a gene linked to our cancers, there wasn't anything we could do about it. At that point, doctors hadn't yet discovered the surgeries, medications, and diagnostic tests that can help manage a person's risk for inherited cancer. Now there are ways to reduce the risk involved in most hereditary cancer syndromes. I'll talk about the ways you can reduce your risk later in the book; each is a strategy that can help prevent biology from becoming destiny.

There was a lot of cancer in my family—and it was everywhere. I particularly wondered about my father's side of the family. Grumpy, as we all affectionately called my dad, had a tumor of the adrenal gland (called a pheochromocytoma) as well as a lung tumor that had been successfully treated with surgery. My family whispered about how Uncle Jack, Grumpy's brother, had died of cancer, and they quietly noted the unnerving similarity in both brothers' cancers. My aunt Evie, my father's sister, had what everyone was calling ovarian cancer (later, I'd have reason to question that label). And then there were my brother and sister, with, respectively, testicular and breast cancer at young ages. Grammy had been treated for endometrial cancer, and her sister had had breast cancer, though these were common cancers that had occurred relatively late in life. From my point of view as a doctor in training (a.k.a. a rookie), these illnesses on Grammy's side were red herrings, nothing that might signify a mutant gene at work.

I couldn't put all the cancers in the paternal line into a clear picture. Were they caused by a mutation? Did I have a mutation, too? I didn't know of any way to connect adrenal, ovarian, testicular, and breast cancers. They're not linked to a known cancer syndrome. But with so much cancer in the family, I also didn't have a reason to stop worrying.

And then, suddenly, I did: A few weeks after I'd settled into my new Brookline condo on the edge of Boston, I received a letter from the hospital that had treated Bea for her cancer two years before. Our entire family had enrolled in a genetic study there, and the counselor wanted to let us know that the scientists saw no reason to believe that Bea's cancer was due to a genetic predisposition. The cancers in my family had been just bad luck. I wasn't at an increased risk for cancer after all, and neither were Bea's children. That August, I flew out to Alex's wedding and celebrated with the rest of the family.

I returned from the wedding just before midnight on Sunday. I dropped my backpack, stray books, and running gear in the foyer, more than ready to get some sleep before returning to the wards in the morning. I fell into bed but noticed the light blinking on my answering machine. I hit the button and heard the message:

Hello, Theo. It's Mom here. I didn't want to interfere with the wedding, but I wanted you to know that a couple of weeks ago I had a mammogram and a biopsy. They found cancer. I'm supposed to have surgery. Before that happens, I want you to have a discussion with the doctor. OK? Don't tell anyone.

Another cancer in the family. Amid my concern for Grammy, I reminded myself that breast cancer in seventy-something women is fairly common. This was clearly a case of sporadic, not inherited, cancer.

In fact, Grammy did have a garden-variety, estrogen receptor–positive cancer—the kind that older women tend to have and that is far more treatable than the swiftly progressing breast cancer that tends to strike women at a younger age. With this news, I reviewed the breast cancer literature and was impressed by the results doctors were getting with a relatively new drug called tamoxifen. The studies of tamoxifen were well controlled and had been performed on lots of patients, which meant the good results the studies reported were probably caused by the drug's positive effects and not by chance or bias. Tamoxifen was not even designed to treat breast cancers; it was developed by Arthur Walpole in the 1960s as a contraceptive to block estrogen's actions. Powerful observations and strong collaborations led to the development of tamoxifen as the first targeted cancer treatment. It has saved the lives of hundreds of thousands of women with breast cancer. Even back then I realized immediately that Grammy's chances were excellent.

The next day, one day before Grammy was scheduled for surgery, the phone rang again.

This call was from Bea, calling from Omaha:

My doctor thinks that the sciatica we talked about on the way to the airport is breast cancer. It's returned. It's in my bone marrow. Will you talk with my doctor? Don't tell anybody.

More cancer. Worse, cancer that had metastasized deep into Bea's bones. More secrets, too. My mother and sister were now carrying dueling breast cancer diagnoses, and I was supposed to keep both illnesses to myself.

As I would learn over the years, cancer secrecy can have its roots in problems that feel difficult to manage: anxiety, protectiveness of oneself and others, shame, or a deeply ingrained cultural habit of keeping a lid on health issues. My family has experienced all these brands of cancer secrecy, but the situation I was in now felt different. Both Grammy and Bea had asked me to keep quiet, and of course I wanted to respect their desire for privacy. After all, *I* wasn't the one who was sick. Weren't they the ones who should make the decisions about who knows about their illness? Yet they didn't really seem that concerned about their privacy. Mostly, they said that they didn't want anyone else in the family to be worried.

When I returned Grammy's call on Monday to discuss her situation, she said, "I'll be fine! It's practically normal to get breast cancer at my age! Talking about it is just going to make everyone worry about me. I wouldn't have told you except that you're a doctor."

"I don't want people to bother themselves about me," Bea said. "Let's wait until we know more before saying anything."

I asked a colleague to join me for a strategy dinner to get his objective take on the situation. What should I do? Why doesn't anyone want to cause worry? Why doesn't anyone want to be a bother? Why are they so concerned about everyone else at a time when they have good reason to worry about themselves?

My colleague helped me by taking my attention away from the "why" questions, pointing out that these were not likely to yield any real answers or shake loose any helpful insights that would help me make a decision. Instead, he walked me through the different possible outcomes of my mother's and sister's treatments. He asked me to imagine the potential damage that secrets could cause, depending on which outcomes came true.

It's challenging to survey your mother's and sister's cancers and think about all the possible scenarios, including the worst ones. I started with the most hopeful: If both Grammy's and Bea's treatments went smoothly and successfully, I could easily preserve their secrets. But I reminded myself of the mental calculations I'd been making about the cancers in our family. If somehow it turned out that Bea's old hospital was wrong and that our cancers were inherited after all, I'd be withholding information that could help us all understand more about our risk for cancer. And if Grammy had a stroke on the operating table—this is a rare complication of surgery, but nevertheless possible—my brothers and sister might discover they had missed their last chance to speak with her. Bea, on the other hand, had a treatment plan that looked very difficult, and the prognosis for her metastatic breast cancer wasn't good. If I didn't tell my family about her illness now, when would they learn about it?

So I spilled the beans. I called Bea to tell her about our mother's cancer—and explained that I couldn't keep family health secrets, including hers. Then I called Grammy and had a similar conversation. I expected them to be horrified or angry, but here's what I discovered: Neither of them really wanted secrecy. They were mostly just overwhelmed at the thought of having to hash out the details of their illness with every family member—this was on top of being sick and having to make choices about their treatments. I offered to serve as medical translator and family communications officer, an admittedly ironic job for someone who'd originally been entrusted with a double set of secrets. (It's not for nothing that my family nickname is Aunt Blabby.) Partly as a result of this experience, whenever I have a patient who is hesitant to talk about cancer with his or her family, I suggest appointing someone close who can attend medical visits and speak with family members on the patient's behalf. This person doesn't have to be a medical professional, just someone who is good at asking questions, hunting down information, and patiently explaining complex situations. This strategy keeps communication flowing and avoids the kind of secrecy that isn't really secrecy—it's just discomfort with transmitting information that can be a mix of the technical and emotional. There's a lot about inheriting a vulnerability to cancer that is inevitably hard. When it's within your power to make things easier, seize the opportunity. It's not difficult to dispel this particular kind of secrecy, and the information you share could eventually save the lives of people you love.

It was only a couple of weeks before it became clear to all of us that Bea was not going to make it beyond a month. We all dropped our daily lives and traveled to be with her and her family. With one exception: Grammy's tumor was being treated with radiation and the treatment tied her to home five days a week. She was to come on the weekend.

A few days after I arrived at Bea's hospital, the cancer was taking over her liver. I remained vigilant, hoping that somehow I could help Bea recover. Miraculous recoveries were a pattern in the family; we had a tradition of big illnesses ending up "all better." But Bea slipped into the final phases of her disease. Grumpy made a distress call to Grammy from Bea's bedside. She got on the next plane to Omaha, and to hell with her radiation. But by then, Bea was gone. Watching Grammy take in the sight of Bea was overwhelming. Because her daughter could not survive cancer, my mother would be a reluctant survivor herself. These sights can change a person. They can motivate you to do things you couldn't have imagined.

Charting Your Family's Health History

Once again, I dropped my backpack in the doorway as I returned home to my Brookline condo. This time, though, I reentered my life transformed. I'd been a serious student of medicine and science, but now I was a woman with a quest, and I was going to shed all things extraneous to my goal. I broke off my relationship because it was not part of my new mission. Marriage and children, I decided, would have to be postponed. Already my hospital rotations were helping me gain a better understanding of diseases, especially cancer. I decided that I'd focus all my energy on these career plans and ultimately participate in the identification and analysis of the genes that were running through families with hereditary cancers.

In the meantime I had a more immediate task. Despite what Bea's old hospital had reported to me, I had reason again to wonder if cancer was passing through our family via our genes. This time, I wasn't going to merely think through my family history in my head. I took out a pencil and, for the first time, attempted to work out our family's cancer story on paper. I drew a family pedigree, which is a tool I'd learned as a graduate student for tracking diseases through a family's generations and branches. At the time, pencil to paper was the norm. Today there are numerous Web-based programs that can help you draw your family's pedigree.

In a pedigree, the ethnic heritage of each major branch of the family is noted at the top. Then each generation is shown by a line, like a branch on a tree. The generations are given Roman numerals, and every person in a generation receives an Arabic numeral. Squares represent men and circles represent women, and their current ages, or age at the time of death, are written above the shapes. A horizontal line between two shapes indicates a marriage or union, and a vertical line that descends from a horizontal line leads to the offspring. Siblings are joined by a horizontal line. If a person has died, there is a diagonal slash through the square or circle, and the cause of death is written underneath. Everyone who has had cancer gets a mark inside their shape; the kind of mark is determined by the kind of cancer they've had. You can see the standard marks for some common cancers in the pedigree on the facing page, but not all cancers have standardized pedigree markings. What's important is that you use a clear key at the bottom of the pedigree, so that other people can interpret the way you've chosen to code your family's history.

At this point, here's what my family's pedigree looked like to me (see page 37). It covered four generations.

If you have any questions at all about the cancer in your family, performing this exercise is a must. I recommend drafting a pedigree

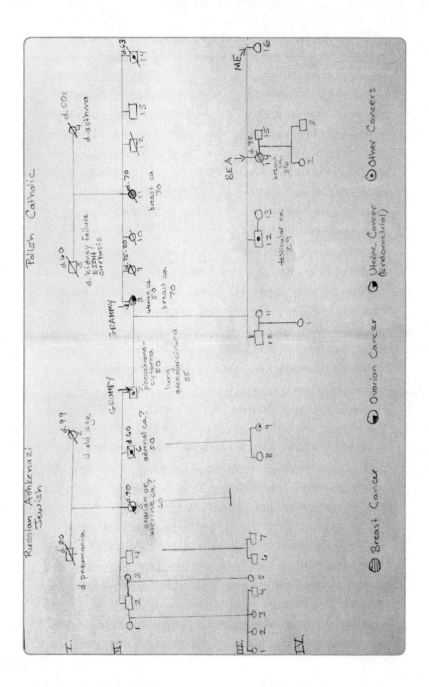

right now. If that's not possible, draft one as soon as you can. The pedigree I drew shows four generations of direct descendants; it's best to include as many generations and family members as possible. If you can go back for more generations than I could, then do! If you have cousins, half-siblings, or mystery relatives of unknown parentage, include them, too—even if you have to make special branches of the pedigree just for them. On paper or on a screen, you're more likely to see patterns you didn't notice before, or to understand where it is you need more information. If you decide to work with a genetic counselor later, that work will be useless without a pedigree that is as complete as possible.

What if you create a pedigree only to find that it's incomplete? Don't lose heart. Most of us have trouble filling in the spaces—and that's the best-kept secret in the business. You can see that I couldn't fill in a few pieces of information on my pedigree at the time. Doctors, genetic counselors, and the writers of websites and pamphlets will advise you to create a family pedigree (they might use a different phrase, like "fill out your family tree") before taking a next step, like seeing a doctor or genetic counselor. But getting the family information to put into the pedigree is the hard part. So I'll say it now: Expect blank spots in your pedigree. Expect family members to make it hard for you to get crucial medical information, even if they do so in the nicest way. Expect to hear stories about an illness that are puzzling or contradictory. The next chapters will help you find effective ways to address these problems.

I understand the difficulties that so many patients experience when filling out a family pedigree because I ran into them myself. At the time I prepared the pedigree on page 37, I once again saw a family tree that was filled with cancer. Still, it didn't follow a pattern that I could link to a particular genetic syndrome. What I didn't know then was that there were things I didn't know.

Chapter Three

Taking a Family History:
Dealing with Silence,
Dealing with Drama

LONG BEFORE THAT AFTERNOON in my Brookline condo when I first tried to work on my family's cancer pedigree—before Bea's cancer first appeared and before it ever crossed my mind that my family might have inherited a predisposition to cancer—I realized that my family was not going to make it easy for me to learn the truth about their background, medical or otherwise. My family had secrets.

This secrecy was ironic, because Grammy (my mother) has always valued honesty. She and Grumpy (my father) raised my brothers, sister, and me in the 1960s and '70s, an era when America was fascinated with things that were not quite authentic: TV dinners, plastic furniture, Nixon. Grammy clearly thought this trend was in poor taste. She wanted everything to be *real.* She insisted on real wood logs for the fireplace; on trudging for hours through the Michigan snow to chop down a real fir Christmas tree; on having children who would be useful adults; on making sure that we always told the truth.

Unfortunately for me, telling the truth would have meant confronting my parents with some uncomfortable facts. At age eight,

I was flunking elementary school and trying to charm my way through violin lessons without practicing. My older siblings—Bea, Alex, and Tony—were accomplished musicians, athletes, and students. But I had zero ambition. I didn't want to hurt Grammy by telling her that I hated school and violin, so . . . I lied.

I was a talented liar. For fun, I'd hide Grumpy's shoes at night, and in the morning he'd rant about his missing shoes. Then, when his back was turned, I'd put his shoes in a place that he'd already looked for them. After a few minutes, I'd play the hero by miraculously finding his "lost" shoes. When Grammy would ask me whether I'd practiced violin while she was out at the store, I'd tell her, with a straight face, that "it was just scales for an hour—but enjoyable nevertheless." As my mother liked to say, I had "underdeveloped forearms and an overdeveloped imagination."

Fortunately, I had an ally in creative fibbing: Uncle Jack. A few times a year, Grammy and Grumpy drove us from our home in Kalamazoo, Michigan, in our old blue Dodge station wagon to see relatives on the East Coast. We always stopped in New Jersey to pay a visit to Uncle Jack, my father's brother, and Jack's wife, Aunt Gladys. Jack and Gladys's mansion was the opposite of our plain, 1950s-style ranch home. Jack and Gladys had a grand foyer, complete with a walk-in closet; their dining room boasted a long, sleek table that I'd never seen in use; and they had such a big yard that although I ran to each window in the house, I could never see all the way to a neighbor's home. Their living room was lined with mirrors, and I sometimes wondered, was I in the real living room, or in one of the living rooms reflected back to me? Their fireplace was deliciously fake—no fire, no smoke, just plastic logs.

Jack and I would sit on the couch of his family room and spin stories.

He told me about how his maternal grandparents, Hyman and Motlu Silverstein, had probably been subjects of the Russian emperor just before they'd immigrated with their nine children to

New Jersey in 1911. Jack himself didn't know much about his paternal line, but he did tell me that he had been born with the name Jacob Rosenblum. In 1939, when Jack wanted to apply for a teaching job in Camden, New Jersey, a friend advised him that with a name like Jacob Rosenblum, he would be rejected. He needed a good "Anglo-Saxon" name. So Jack's parents, my grandparents, changed the family name to Ross and Jack's first name to William. Jack got the job.

Jack told me how my dad (a Russian-Italian Jew) and my mother (raised as a Polish Catholic) eloped, got married in a Baptist church, and moved to the Midwest to start fresh. Their families forgave them, Jack said, because my dad was a lucky charm and my mom was mesmerizing.

My parents? Glamorous? This was news to me.

"You know," Jack said, passing a hand through his bushy hair, "your mom loves good music and nice art. And there's something mysterious about her background. It wouldn't surprise me if your mother was descended from Slavic royalty. *Your* great-grandfather could have been *my* grandfather's emperor."

"No *shit*," I said.

The word "shit" was a joke between us, and something of a secret password. Jack had explained to me that "shit" was an unusually flexible word that could express almost any thought.

"Let's shoot the shit," Jack might say to me as we settled onto the couch.

"Sure," I'd say. "I've been trapped in the car for hours with a bunch of dipshits."

"Bet you've been going apeshit."

We both enjoyed the volley. One time I laughed so hard that I peed all over his couch, which only made him laugh harder. No one had to know about my accident, he assured me.

"Who's to say what's true?" he'd counsel. "Who's to say that *your* truth is always right?" If you had to lie because it would protect somebody from unnecessary pain (including yourself), Jack was all for it. I looked forward to visiting his house the way a prisoner anticipates release.

Then Jack disappeared. The last time I saw him was on a visit in 1974, when I was eleven years old. Instead of hanging out in the family room, I sat around the kitchen table with Aunt Gladys and the rest of my family. My parents told me that Jack would come out of his bedroom to say hello to all of us, but he didn't say a word. He just shuffled into the kitchen in his bathrobe, his eyes uncharacteristically averted, and waved sideways before sliding back to his room. The adults shook their heads, murmuring, *all he does is smoke and sleep*. On the next visit, there was no Jack, no explanation.

I knew that Jack had died, of course, and without anyone directly telling me not to speak of his death, I also knew that the topic was off-limits. Things felt secret, a bit shameful. The adults' grief was real but hidden in "low talk"—in whispers and in conversations that took place after I was supposed to be asleep. Once Grammy had a long conversation on the phone with Aunt Gladys. She hung up, sighed, and said, "Gladys speaks so softly now. It's as if half of her followed him."

I remembered Jack's lessons in half-truths and decided to ignore all the things that the adults weren't saying. I thought we might all be a little happier if I put my mind toward success—or, at least, a facsimile thereof. I consulted Bea (known respectfully as "Bea Wiz"; before Jack disappeared, he had helped me nickname everybody we knew). I asked her how to avoid flunking out of seventh grade and how to appear more ambitious. She laid out a short but effective plan. The first step was to study a school subject for ten minutes a day, every day, first thing in the morning. I was to follow this with fifteen minutes of violin practice after school. After that I was free to do whatever.

One of my favorite "whatevers" involved Gilda Radner, a fellow Michigander. She was just making it big on the comedy scene. After

I did my work, sometimes Bea Wiz and I listened to Radner on the radio. On Saturdays the entire family tried to stay awake for Radner's *Saturday Night Live* Roseanne Roseannadanna sketches. I followed Bea Wiz's recipe of study, violin, and "whatever" precisely, and it worked pretty well. My grades improved. I started to play in tune. And when I didn't, I just followed Roseanne Roseannadanna's lead: *Never mind,* I'd say to myself in Roseanne's pinched little voice, and try again.

Cancer secrecy was typical of the time. Cancer just wasn't discussed, and especially not a death from cancer. Even children were encouraged to sink their grief into activity. To a certain extent, this strategy worked, at least for me. I studied violin seriously enough to drop out of high school and attend music school at Indiana University. Privately, I wanted to be a doctor, maybe because of a curiosity about cancer secrecy. (Who doesn't want to know about secrets?) Eventually, I went to college and then on to my graduate training as a physician-scientist.

For my family, though, and plenty of others, this cultural secrecy about cancer meant that important medical history got covered up and sometimes lost altogether. In our clinic, patients often say things like "We never talked about health problems," or "Cancer was something my parents would have never discussed." In a way, these patients are the lucky ones. They realize that there might be some question marks in the cancer pedigree, some cancers in the family that they haven't been told about. But many people don't even know that there are family secrets in the first place.

One of our patients, for example, told us that her mother had hidden her own diagnosis and treatment for breast cancer when she was forty-six. This is a crucial fact for a cancer pedigree, because when breast cancer appears in a woman who is younger than fifty, it's considered a red flag for an inherited cancer syndrome. But it was the 1960s, a time when cancer just wasn't talked about—and when doctors didn't know about inherited cancer syndromes. It wasn't until years later, when the mother's cancer returned, that finally she told her children. If her mother hadn't relapsed, her children would never have known that there was a secret cancer. Sometimes cancer secrecy has influenced the way doctors practiced. Years after Gilda Radner died of ovarian cancer, her husband, Gene Wilder, told the press that Radner's cancer had gone undiagnosed for a long time. When Radner went to doctors with her symptoms, no one asked her whether she had a family cancer history. (This was the 1980s, when it was established that ovarian cancer can run in families.) If her doctors had known that Radner's grandmother, aunt, and cousin each had the disease, they might have considered a cancer diagnosis earlier, and she might have received treatment faster.

We've gotten better about being open with medical histories, especially cancer. Betty Ford's disclosure of her treatment for breast cancer in 1974 and Radner's description of her difficulty in getting her ovarian cancer properly diagnosed in 1986 helped propel cancer out of the dark. But misinformation and missing information from that earlier era is still a problem for those of us trying to fill in our cancer pedigrees. And there are plenty of people who still keep cancer secrets today. I see it all the time in the clinic. If you don't think there are any cancer secrets in your family, consider this: A study published by Phuong L. Mai and her colleagues in the *Journal of the National Cancer Institute* reported that when people disclose their cancer histories, those histories are usually inaccurate. The investigators asked more than a thousand Connecticut residents about cancers in their first- and second-degree relatives and then checked that information against data in registries, Medicare databases, death certificates, and other health records. Of those cancer histories, 40 to 75 percent contained errors, with reports of breast cancer being most accurate and lung cancer being least accurate. For example, there is frequent confusion whether a relative's "lung" cancer originated in the lung or had metastasized to the lung.

That day in my Brookline condo when I tried to draw my family's pedigree, I realized that I needed to learn more about why Jack died. Over the years, I'd discovered a bit more about his illness. Ten years after Jack's death, when I was twenty-one, Grumpy had been diagnosed with a pheochromocytoma, a tumor of the adrenal medulla. (The adrenal medulla is the inside part of the adrenal gland; it secretes adrenaline-type hormones.) The older members of the family murmured of the "symmetry" between Jack's cancer and Grumpy's. To my untrained ears—I had not yet been to medical school—it sounded as if Jack had also had an adrenal cancer. I'd been going on that assumption ever since. But as I looked at the pedigree eight years later, now with the eyes of a medical intern, I started to doubt that assumption. Adrenal cancer is rare; its appearance among the other cancers within my family sat far outside any known pattern. As I stared at the paper on which I'd drawn the family pedigree, I also zeroed in on the little wedge that represented the cancer of my dad's sister, Aunt Evie. At around the same time Grumpy was being treated for cancer, Aunt Evie was diagnosed with what some in the family called "ovarian" cancer. But as I sat and looked at the paper, I remembered that there were other family members who described her cancer as "endometrial." I was now far enough along in my training to know that cancers in the female reproductive system are frequently mixed up. Understanding this difference is important, because each of these cancers can be signals of different inherited cancer syndromes. If I could dredge up the truth about Jack's and Evie's cancers, I might find that the pedigree fit a known pattern of inherited cancer.

I also realized that getting to the truth about our cancers was going to be difficult. It's not that my family was harboring a Gothic secret (to my knowledge). There were no hidden dungeons with skeletons chained to the wall, no children who had been locked away in the attic. It was *just cancer*. But still . . . we all had an unspoken agreement not to talk about the cancers from that generation, and we'd abided by that agreement for so long. Not talking about it was as tightly woven into our family as was music and respect for family elders. Raising the topic could disturb the family's ecosystem, upset its balance. Bringing up the subject would be awkward. As the youngest and therefore the lowest on the family totem pole, I thought I was unlikely to succeed. I was glad that I, as a medical intern, had an excuse for not probing too far into what felt like forbidden territory. I was going to be a doctor, after all, and a researcher. I needed to put all my focus into my education and my patients. At least, that's what I told myself.

I didn't realize it then, but my dilemma is a common one. When families aren't talking openly about cancer, how do you get an accurate family history? A similar question applies to families with hazy medical memories, families with estrangements and conflicts, and people who are adopted. Over the years, I've learned some helpful tools and work-arounds.

Genogram to the Rescue

Imagine that you've drawn your family's pedigree on a whiteboard. You've made your circles for women and squares for men, with lines to represent unions and births. But now imagine that some of those solid lines transform, before your eyes, into dotted ones. Or they become zigzags. Some get broken up. Some double up, so that instead of one line there are two running parallel.

What's just happened?

The official name for the new configuration on that whiteboard is genogram. A genogram is a lot like a family cancer pedigree, but it doesn't look only at cancer history. A genogram is a tool used in psychology, and its main concern is emotional. Unlike the fact-based cancer pedigree, a genogram has an additional vocabulary of shapes and lines to express the ways families act when they're under pressure. When it feels hard to ask for information about family health, or hard to get it, a genogram can help you understand why.

To create a genogram, start with your cancer pedigree. If you haven't been able to completely fill out your pedigree, don't worry—just do the best you can. If you're unsure about any family members or cancers, make a note of it on the pedigree. Then, once you've got your pedigree drawn, add in features that characterize the emotional quality of the relationships. For example:

Harmonic

Draw a straight line between two people to indicate a harmonious relationship.

Close

Two straight lines between two people indicate a very close relationship.

Distant

A broken line indicates a distant relationship.

Conflicted

Two broken lines mean that there's conflict in the relationship.

Cut Off/Estranged

A broken line with two slash marks indicates two people who aren't speaking.

Hostile

A wavy or zigzag line means that the relationship is hostile.

You can use other signs if you want to, or describe different emotional states; the examples above are here to give you the basic idea and to get you started. The concept behind the genogram is that families are systems—and when families experience anxiety, the system feels unstable. Family members then seek out stability by reacting in predictable but troublesome ways. Because cancer naturally causes so much anxiety, it's common to find these painful patterns at play when you try to unearth your family history. This is a reason that apparently straightforward questions like "I'm filling out our family medical history. Can you help me?" can feel as forbidden as asking, "Why don't you and Aunt Jane visit each other anymore?"

A genogram makes patterns in the family more visible. Some of them include:

- CONFLICT: When people feel anxious, they may look for fights. Is there someone in your family who may have had cancer, or who may have information about another member's illness, but who has such a large chip on his or her shoulder that you're afraid to ask? Are you connected by two dotted lines?

- DISTANCE: Does your family tend to handle problems by going silent? This coping pattern can masquerade as forgetfulness ("Oh, I must not have seen your email"), superiority ("I'm not going to waste my time by having this conversation"), or protectiveness ("You're too young to worry about all that stuff"). When I told myself that I was too busy to ask why Uncle Jack died, and that it would be no use in asking anyway, I was practicing a form of distance, too. A dotted line connected me to Aunt Gladys, Uncle Jack's widow. Gladys would be connected to Jack with two straight lines as they were, to my knowledge, close and not conflicted.

- ESTRANGEMENT: If there are people in your family you're not allowed to talk to, or whole branches of the family that don't speak to each other, you may be dealing with people who don't know any other way to cope with emotional tension. Grammy, for example, stopped speaking to her brother Joe after she left for college, and now his history is mysterious to us all. I met him once when I was very little, when Grammy took me to see the house in Philadelphia she had grown up in. Though her brother, Uncle Joe, still lived there, we didn't stay long. I found that curious but didn't have the guts to ask any good questions about it. As we walked out of her childhood home, she murmured that she'd never speak to him again; on our genogram there's a dotted line with two slash marks in the middle disconnecting Grammy and Uncle Joe. (Of course, some people decide to end contact with a family member because of an abusive situation. This decision can be a mature, lifesaving choice.)

* TRIANGULATION: When two people focus on a third person as "the problem," a triangle occurs. If you decide to ask about cancer history, other family members may pull together to grouse about the trouble you're causing. That triangulation makes them feel less anxious and more stable. But it can make *you* feel uncomfortable.

The genogram that I'm asking you to draw now is meant to help you gather information about your family history of cancer, so characterize your relationships and mark up the genogram with this goal in mind. If your aunt is close to all her nieces and nephews but clams up when it comes to cancer, mark that relationship as "distant," just for the purpose of talking about your family history. Mark the genogram according to the current state of the relationship, not how it felt in the past. If your grandmother and sister were completely estranged for a couple of years but have found their way back to a good relationship, your genogram should read as "harmonic" or even "close."

Your genogram can expose your family's favorite ways to manage cancer anxiety—and most families participate in at least a few of them. Cancer makes most of us scared. It brings up painful losses. It reminds us of death and suffering. Some people feel shame about illness, especially if it's associated with a lifestyle choice like smoking. People who are usually rational can be secretly superstitious about cancer, feeling that if they don't talk about it, cancer won't touch them. And some people are very uncomfortable sharing information about parts of their bodies—breasts, uterus, testicles, ovaries, prostate—that are usually kept private. Your genogram can reveal a general trend of managing cancer anxiety through distance (lots of broken lines), or emotional cutoff (broken lines and slash marks), or triangulation (often seen when two people have the double lines of a close bond and a third person is cut off in some way).

These patterns can make it hard to get a family history. It can feel awkward, forbidden, or even impossible. If I had known about genograms back when I was struggling to complete my family's pedigree, I would have seen a pattern of closeness, but also of distance. Maybe that explains why both Bea and my mom reacted to their cancers by confiding in me—and then asking me to keep quiet. Maybe that's why Jack's cancer felt so submerged and secret. I also would have seen another pattern of silence: I seemed to know a lot more about Grumpy's side of the family than I did about Grammy's, and there was more emotional contact with Grumpy's family, too.

Psychology offers some suggestions for reaching out and getting the truth, even when the patterns of anxiety are making things feel tense and difficult. Jeffrey Kendall, Psy.D., a professor and clinical leader of Oncology Supportive Services at UT Southwestern, helps our patients with their own reactions to illness and to have difficult conversations with their families. He notes that every family's system of function and dysfunction is different, so there are an infinite number of ways to get to the truth, some more efficient than others, and all dependent on the context of the family's system.

Kendall says that the number-one factor that gets in the way of conversations about family history and genetics is a general lack of health literacy: "Genetics, in particular, is complicated. People—patients and professionals—don't fully understand genetics. Why should we expect family members to get it with a single conversation or email exchange?" He goes on to say, "Letting patients and their family members know that this is a difficult topic for everybody is a good first step. The issues of blame, guilt, shame, and fear that come with having an illness or a gene mutation can come from a lack of understanding—from a lack of health literacy."

When Kendall is sitting in his office with somebody we've sent to him for guidance on difficult family conversations, he tells them that there are three parts to the conversation:

1. The before;
2. The during; and
3. The after.

For the "before," Kendall tells patients to use him, a genetic counselor, or a doctor to clarify and then write down the information they are going to discuss. He advises patients to write short sentences, which will help them better understand what they want to say. And what they want to say will also depend on how the family system is structured. This is where the family system, as illustrated on the genogram, comes in. If the daughter plans to talk with a very emotional mother with whom she is not close, telling the mother that the information will help both of them is not that useful. But if she tells the mother it will help her grandson, the mother may be more open to an information exchange. On the other end of the spectrum, if the planned conversation is with her beloved twin brother who is also an engineer, that brother will likely want to learn all he can to help himself as well as his sister. Kendall also coaches our patients in ways to calm themselves prior to these discussions, including taking deep breaths, meditating, reading their short sentences to themselves, and replacing thoughts about past errors with hopes for the future.

For the "during" part, Kendall recommends emphasizing and explaining why the information matters for the future. He suggests focusing on building collaboration, speaking in short sentences (no rambling), encouraging questions, and encouraging emotions.

What happens in the "after" period will depend on what happened in the "during." If the parent feigns a lack of knowledge and responds with "I don't remember," or if the parent is angry and responds with "You're being difficult. Why do you bring this stuff up? Go away," patients can still follow up. Kendall offers this advice: Don't expect the reactions to be simple or predictable. Do all you can to be prepared, but remember that you can't control all that happens in the "during" phase. "After" is a matter of consolidation, writing the information down, and following up as best you can by letting family members know what you found out and how that impacts the family.

In the very common situation in which a branch of the family is estranged, Kendall notes, patients may need to prepare more (meditate longer or consider bringing in an ally) and do what they can to guide the conversation or communication focused on the future— because, of course, the past is where the estrangement began. Kendall says, "Preparation has to match the difficulty and needs of the actual conversation." By focusing on the future, you "get away from the sources of silence, lies, and tension in the family." As an example, he suggests saying, "No matter what the past was, this is what we need to do to move our family forward and protect ourselves." Families tend to obsess on the history of their mistakes. This is what builds the foundation of that family's system (illustrated by the genogram), which was considered as part of the "before" preparations. Whether to have the conversation one-on-one or within a group depends on the family. Kendall says, "Sometimes bringing in the eighty-five-year-old grandmother whom everybody respects as an ally can be of help. And if her presence helps you stay relaxed, that's a bonus."

Carolyn Daitch, Ph.D., the director of the Center for the Treatment of Anxiety Disorders in Farmington Hills, Michigan, has additional advice for family conversations about cancer history. She suggests acknowledging the other person's worries. This can be especially helpful when talking with someone you're generally close to but who is distant on the subject of cancer. Daitch recommends an opener that goes something like this:

This might be hard for you to talk about, and I totally get why it might be. But I'm wondering if there would be a good time when I can ask you some questions about our family that would be very helpful to me.

"We're always on safer ground," Daitch says, "if we can imagine the other person's feelings—reluctance, fear, or resistance—and acknowledge them. It also increases the likelihood that the person will want to prove you wrong."

When someone is hesitant to share information, Daitch recommends using this line:

A part of you knows that this is the right thing to do.

Say this in a kind, encouraging voice, not a dark and threatening one. Daitch says, "It meets people on a higher level."

Of course, there is no single method of communication that is always right, and there's not even one that's always wrong. I think of approaching families about sensitive subjects in the way that I think about talking to colleagues or trainees in the lab. I try to treat everyone based on his or her individual temperament. Is there a graduate student who needs positive feedback to feel invigorated? Is there a new employee who works better under a rigid two-by-four management style? What helps each one make better decisions, and what causes them to freeze up? No one in the lab is quite like anyone else in the lab, and the same goes for all the members of your family. It's worth taking stock of each person, respecting and accepting who they are, and working with that knowledge. This work might be stressful, but often it's good stress, the kind that eventually leads to both more openness and more closeness.

Your genogram might help you spot the person with the most knowledge in the family—this is the person with lots of double lines that connect to other people—and you can always try asking that person to help you with your project. For example, Bea was the oldest and smartest of the four kids in my family. While she was alive, she was the one people trusted with family information; she was also the one who could remember it accurately. I bet she would have known the truth about Aunt Evie's cancer, and I wish I'd asked her more about Evie before they both died.

To the recommendations above, I'll add some more ways my patients have successfully gathered family medical information:

- Ask at family reunions or weddings, where almost everyone you might want to talk with is corralled in one place. You don't need to make your request over a megaphone. Just go quietly from family member to family member and chat over the potato salad or appetizers.
- Talk to family members at funerals and memorial services. While these events can be stressful, they're often times of greater authenticity and communication. Use your judgment and consider asking questions if the time seems right.
- Tracking down death certificates for family members might also help. They are publically available and can be obtained in person from the Department of Vital Statistics in any state, or from vitalchek.com.

- Use social media to locate estranged branches of the family. If you don't have an urgent need to know your history, you might slowly build up a relationship through messages and "likes"—and then ask your questions.
- When one family member isn't talking, ask different relatives. In other words, go around the mountain if you can't go over it. Your parents—even if you're middle-aged—may still be in the old habit of protecting you from unpleasant information. Uncles, aunts, and cousins may be more willing to talk.
- Don't let the family judge whether medical information is accurate. One of our patients was told by a relative that there was no cancer in the family but that there was a weird instance when a doctor "claimed" that her uncle had breast cancer. Of course, the man really *had* died of breast cancer, and this crucial piece of information meant that our patient needed to be tested for BRCA1 and BRCA2 mutations.
- Don't just ask your family about the things you're unsure of; also double-check the things you think you know. You might have heard people saying that your aunt had brain cancer, but asking something like "Are you sure she definitely had a diagnosis of brain cancer? How did you find out?" might reveal that they are simply repeating something they've heard thirdhand. Try to find someone with direct knowledge of the diagnosis.
- See a genetic counselor. The counselor can help you contact family members and, with the family members' permission, the counselor can take the baton and ask key questions and work to acquire medical records for each family member. If both you and your family member agree, your counselor will even contact your family on your behalf. (In chapter 5, I'll explain more about genetic counselors, what they do, and how to find one.)

- Always write down what you learn, to guard against your own anxiety and simple forgetfulness.

It helps to think of yourself as part detective, part mad scientist, part master manipulator. The most startling example of this combination that I know of is a patient who booked a flight with her mother and then used their time in the air to get her mother drunk on vodka tonics and pelt her with questions. (She discovered that there was a hidden family history of ovarian cancer.) Not a psychologist-approved method, probably, but the underlying message here is that sometimes you just have to do whatever it takes.

The results of your family research won't always be what you want them to be. If you can't put a label on every cancer or death in your genogram or pedigree, know that this is a common situation— and if all you've done is identify what you *don't* know, you've still made a great leap forward. And your investigation is never over. Family conversations can continue. With time you'll learn more and more information—as long as you keep your ears and eyes open.

Fuzzy Facts: When the Family's Cancer Truth Is Lost to History

I never did learn much about Jack's cancer. Everyone called his disease "adrenal cancer," but laypeople use the phrase imprecisely. The most common "adrenal cancers" are actually tumors that start in another place, like in the lung, and then spread through the blood to the adrenal gland. Then again, there are rare cancers—like pheochromocytomas, the one Grumpy had—that originate in the adrenal gland and overproduce the adrenaline hormones that induce anxiety. Other primary adrenal gland cancers called adrenocortical cancers, also rare, can overproduce steroid hormones that lead to manic personality changes. It was possible, I mused, that Jack's colorful personal style and his fascination with words that held shock value were due to hormonal imbalances.

But that was only the magical thinking of my overdeveloped imagination. There are no data on Uncle Jack's tumor. I sought records from the hospital in New Jersey that cared for him, but it was too late. The records had been destroyed. This was a necessity for many hospitals with limited storage space in the pre–electronic record era. Loss of medical records is an unfortunate recurring theme for cancer-in-the-family detectives; sometimes we are left with nothing to go on but the remembered whispers of a diagnosis. With the development of electronic medical records, fewer medical histories will be lost. However, you may encounter a different problem, something along the lines of "HIPAA rules prevent us from sending the records to you," referring to the privacy and security regulations of the Health Insurance Portability and Accountability Act. No matter why you are told that you can't have the records, don't give up easily. If the hospital or doctor's office cites HIPAA, ask whose permission you need to access the records. If they tell you the records are gone, dig around a little bit. Maybe they *are* gone. But maybe they're not. For example, a colleague of mine had some childhood health problems (unrelated to cancer) that led to a yearlong hospitalization. A few years ago, she called the hospital to get the medical records from that time. The person on the other end of the line told her that the records went so far back they certainly had been destroyed. My friend was tempted to lose her temper or hang up. Instead, she explained politely that she was very disappointed and wondered if he was 100 percent sure that they were destroyed. She was surprised when the clerk said, "Well, I'm not 100 percent sure. Let me look and get back to you." She was 100 percent sure she'd never hear from him again. But a day later he called. Many of the records from that time were on microfilm, he explained, and if she gave him a week and a standard processing fee, he'd send them to her.

Back to the question of Jack's cancer diagnosis. Since there are only around three hundred new cases of adrenocortical cancer diagnosed per year in the United States (compared with three hundred thousand new cases of lung cancer), it's likely that our family's memory of Jack having a primary adrenal cancer is incorrect. Jack's tumor was probably a common lung cancer that built a second home in his adrenal gland. In fact, if I were a betting woman, I would say that Jack's cancer was a cigarette-promoted lung cancer that spread to the adrenal glands.

But based on the probabilities, even this bet is, as Jack might say, *bullshit*. When I was younger, Jack taught me that made-up stories can cast a charmed circle around a child, protecting her from adult pressures and stresses. But I was no longer a child. During my training to be a physician-scientist, I learned about the harm that can be done when patients and doctors make up stories to fit what they feel ought to be the truth. My professors taught me that asking careful questions, collecting data, observing a patient's situation, and then re-observing it all with an open mind is the best way to get solid answers. I now try to get the data as my first, second, and third priorities—and only then, with all the available data in hand, do I develop conclusions.

In other words, I learned that my mother was right all along: We have to strive for the truth even when it hurts. We have to be accurate. I want you to think like a detective or a scientist as you collect information about your family's cancers. Thinking like a professional can help you keep your head when things get fuzzy, and cancer is so complicated and weird that I *guarantee* things will get fuzzy.

As for my family history, things stayed fuzzy for a long time. And then, suddenly, they became clearer.

Secret Ethnic Histories

In the years after Bea's death, I finished my residency, oncology fellowship, and postdoctoral research training in Boston, and then I took a job at the University of Michigan, which allowed me to live only a couple of hours away from aging Grammy and Grumpy. I married Sean, a hopelessly handsome kindred spirit and fellow scientist, and we helped raise two adorable toddlers from his previous marriage. We also raised, as we like to joke, several graduate students. In my clinical work, I cared for and treated breast cancer patients. In my lab, we focused on decoding a protein called HIP1 that, when abnormal, causes leukemia and other cancers. In my spare thoughts I dreamed about being able to expand the lab's research to study BRCA1 and BRCA2, as well.

And then I got my melanoma diagnosis. Not long afterward came that snowy winter day, when Sean and I learned that one of my own BRCA1 genes was broken. The pieces of the puzzle finally started coming together. This broken gene was the reason my sister had died—and likely the reason that my brother had developed testicular cancer. It was comforting, after all those years, to finally have an explanation for all the cancer in my family. It was a relief to know that by having prophylactic surgeries, I could, in all likelihood, avoid developing another cancer myself. We had the answer.

Then I paused. What about the extended family? Both my parents had developed multiple cancers. Which side had transmitted the BRCA1 mutation to Bea, Alex, and me? Had the broken gene been passed down through Grammy? Or through Grumpy?

Heather, my genetic counselor, had concluded that the mutation came through my father's side. The BRCA1 gene has several kinds of mutations, and the one I have, the BRCA1 5382insC mutation, is found in families of Ashkenazi Jewish heritage. (It's also found in select other groups of eastern European heritage. However, these groups are less well defined and some of these people may have converted from Judaism during periods of anti-Semitism.)

The Ashkenazi Jewish community provides an example of what population geneticists call the "founder effect." The founder effect occurs when a population is decimated by catastrophic events, such as weather or genocide, or when a small number of people leave one group to establish another (which happened when the Jews migrated from Italy northward through France and into Germany less than eight hundred years ago; other groups that did this were the Hutterites, Amish, French Canadians, Libyan Jews, etc.). "It's a classic founder effect," says Stanford University population geneticist Noah Rosenberg. "A group of perhaps hundreds of people grew into the millions in just a few dozen generations. The genomes of the founders have consequences for the large number of descendants." When a new population arises from a very small number of founders, there is less genetic diversity within the group and even rare forms of genes carried by the founders remain prevalent in successive generations. Gene mutations typically have one of two fates within populations: Strongly deleterious mutations tend not to be passed on and can become increasingly rare or entirely lost. More weakly deleterious mutations, such as BRCA mutations that can cause cancers that arise after the prime childbearing years, tend to become widely dispersed through the population as it grows. When this happens within a small group in which there is intermarriage, there is a greater chance of inheriting certain mutations from not only one of your parents but also from *both* your mother and your father. "Founder populations can have distinctive disease-risk variants or a higher frequency of a widely distributed variant," Rosenberg says. Consequently, in people of Ashkenazi descent, cancer-predisposition syndromes caused by the inheritance of a single mutation from one parent (as happens with BRCA genes and is called autosomal dominant inheritance) are common, as are other inherited diseases that involve the inheritance of a bad copy of the same gene from both parents (called recessive inheritance), like Tay-Sachs disease. Ashkenazi Jews are at a higher risk for both because mutant forms of both genes were present in a small number of the founders.

Other "founder" populations, such as the Amish and the French Canadians of Quebec, also offer classic examples of founder effects. These populations arose from relatively small numbers of original founders and have tended to propagate from intermarriage within the group. They also have increased incidences of certain rare diseases that reflect mutant genes inherited from their founders. The Amish have a *lower* cancer rate than other populations (it's not clear whether to credit genetics or lifestyle), but centuries of intermarriage have made other rare genetic diseases, such as dwarfism and metabolic diseases, more common. The French Canadians of Quebec have specific founder mutations in four breast cancer predisposing genes (BRCA1, BRCA2, PALB2, and CHEK2). Given this information, it's reasonable to offer screening for these founder mutations in all French-Canadian women with breast cancer before the age of fifty. Similarly, if a woman of Ashkenazi Jewish descent is diagnosed with breast cancer before the age of fifty, we test for the three common Ashkenazi Jewish mutations in BRCA1 and BRCA2.

In my family's case, we considered the cancer mystery solved— the case closed. I had the Ashkenazi Jewish mutation, and it was Grumpy's side of the family that was Jewish. Plus, his side had the more pronounced family history of cancer. Jack's cancer, however, posed a problem to this logic. BRCA1 mutations are not associated with either lung or adrenocortical cancer, which were still my best guesses about what Jack had. But the part of me that likes life to be neat and tidy drowned out the part of me that was trained to examine the facts. *Never mind,* I told myself. Jack must have had the mutation, I reasoned, and I began calling members of Grumpy's family, urging them to get tested.

The first relative I called was Grumpy and Jack's youngest brother, Uncle Manny. Manny was understandably concerned about the risk to his five grown children if he tested positive. As a physician himself, Manny understood genetics. He knew right away that if he tested negative, the cancer risk to his children was similar to the risk in the general population (unless of course, their biological mother carried a cancer-causing mutation). Because Manny is a psychiatrist, he was also aware that he needed a genetic counselor to help him sort through the genetic and emotional issues. My genetic counselor, Heather—who had by now earned the title "my beloved genetic counselor"—arranged for Manny to meet with a colleague of hers in Washington, D.C.

While Uncle Manny was waiting to be tested, I was busy thinking about how I could use myself as my first BRCA1 mutant research subject. Then Sean and I made a special trip to Kalamazoo to visit with Grammy to discuss the mutation and its implications for the family. She couldn't understand how Grumpy could have passed a BRCA1 mutation down to his children. She didn't understand how my brother, or any man, could ever have a "breast cancer" mutation.

"Men don't get breast cancer," she insisted.

I explained that, in fact, men *do* get breast cancer and do carry broken breast cancer genes. However, even if men never get cancer, they can still carry genes that predispose their families to cancer and can pass them along to their children. The BRCA mutations predispose people to cancers that are much more frequently observed in women, but the mutations themselves can be carried and passed on by both men and women. I talked to her about family cancer syndromes and about how the mutation I carried could cause not just breast cancer but also ovarian, prostate, and pancreatic cancers, along with melanoma, maybe testicular cancer, and others. Almost certainly, we said, the mutation came from her Jewish husband, who'd had four different cancer diagnoses by the time he'd died.

She was adamant that the cancer couldn't have come from my dad. *She* was the one who'd had breast cancer. *She* was the female. The mutation, she argued, came from her. Sean and I went through the genetics again. It was simple, we said: The mutation came from Grumpy, and each of us kids had a fifty-fifty chance of inheriting it.

Grammy reminded us of the research study our entire immediate family had enrolled in when Bea had been first diagnosed with breast cancer. Given our medical history, we were probably a big, juicy cancer-y feast to the researchers. A perk of participating in the study, which was intended to discover new cancer genes, was that it employed genetic counselors; if any one of us was found to have a cancer mutation, the counselors were supposed to notify all of us. These were the counselors who had sent me a letter just before Bea's cancer came back, saying that our family was in the clear, that we didn't carry a cancer mutation.

"You know," she said, "the research staff had me send in a blood sample."

Huh? I didn't know about that. No one had asked me for a blood sample. Had anyone asked Grumpy?

Grammy had more to say. "Around the time Grumpy was in hospice, they sent me a letter saying that they had some information they'd be willing to share with me if I was interested."

Sean asked to see the letter, and it became clear why she'd filed it away without following up. It read:

We have results from the study to share with you if you are interested. . . . Enclosed is information that will help you to make an informed decision on whether or not to receive your test result. If you are not interested in receiving your test result, please sign and return the enclosed response to our office so that we may update our records regarding your decision.

It was a vague letter. In the context of Grumpy's illness, it had been easy for Grammy to interpret the language as *blah, blah, blah, we are performing a routine duty by sending you a letter that doesn't really mean anything, blah, blah, blah.* Sean began to see red. He realized that the research university had for some time been aware of information that might change the way we thought about our cancer risk. He called a phone number on the form letter, but since it was a Sunday evening, he was put through to an on-call physician who was irritated to be bothered with a genetic question rather than a medical emergency. Sean explained that he just wanted to know what information they had, but nobody was available to speak with him.

My family's genetic history was starting to feel more complicated.

The next day I called the research institution myself, explained the situation, and asked them what the new information was. They were profusely apologetic and said that, yes, my mother had the BRCA1 5382insC mutation. They had discovered it a while back. Yet nobody in my family had found out—because they had sent only a vague form letter to my recently widowed eighty-two-year-old mother. When she had failed to respond, they had not followed up with a phone call. They had not contacted me, even though they had promised to notify family members if there was an increased genetic risk. And I thought that *families* were bad about keeping secrets.

I requested a conversation with the principal investigator of the study. "Sorry, he's not available," they said. I asked them to FedEx all the records they had on our family and then hung up the phone in disbelief. Were there other families that were unaware of test results that might change their medical decisions?

I called my beloved genetic counselor, Heather.

"Grumpy's not the source of the mutation," I said. "Grammy is."

"What?" Heather gasped. I explained what had happened.

"Theo," she said. "I need to ask you a question. Think about it carefully. You and your mother both have the Ashkenazi Jewish cancer mutation. Although it's also found in some non-Jewish families from Slavic countries, I wonder, is it possible your mother is Jewish?"

No, it wasn't possible. Mom was a "good" Polish Catholic girl who had married a Jew and was now agnostic.

But . . . then I remembered what Jack had said about my mom.

There's something mysterious about her background.

It wouldn't surprise me if your mother was descended from Slavic royalty.

I thought about my family's pedigree, about the gaps on my mother's side of the family tree. About how I knew very little about her relatives, other than that both her parents immigrated to Philadelphia from Poland near the end of World War I. When Poland regained independence from Russia in the aftermath of the war, it was the center of the European Jewish world, with one of the world's largest Jewish communities. However, anti-Semitism in the general population may have led many Jews to hide their identities and present themselves as Catholics. Certainly this happened later, as Hitler's power spread through Europe. But this is all speculation. Where Grammy's Jewish genes came from remains a mystery.

Secret ethnic histories are not unusual. Some families hide their ethnicity intentionally, the way Uncle Jack dropped his Jewish names (Rosenblum became Ross) when he realized employers would hold him back in postwar America. Some families lost their identity long ago. This happened in European Jewish families that had to reinvent themselves under Hitler's rule or risk being sent to a concentration camp. Eventually this led to new family traditions, and the ethnic history was lost. This happened to our patient Asha, a successful author and artist in her forties who visited our clinic because her mother had died of breast cancer at age forty-two. When we took her family history, Asha mentioned her proud Irish heritage—and that two of her aunts also had breast cancer at young ages. One died, but the other had survived. We asked if the surviving aunt had taken a genetic test and learned that the aunt had been offered genetic testing and declined it.

So Asha was tested and learned that she has the BRCA1 185delAG mutation, one of the three mutations common to Ashkenazi Jews. Asha, it turned out, was not Irish after all. She was Jewish. When this information was shared with her aunt, the aunt came clean. Asha's mother and her two sisters all knew about their Jewish heritage. During World War II the family converted to Catholicism, made up a story about an Irish homeland, and made a pact never to tell. At the time, the goal was to protect the family, especially the children. Tragically, this kind of protection can have the unintended effect of preventing a family from knowing its cancer risk.

Jerome Price, a family therapist at the Michigan Family Institute, warns that uncovering a hidden ethnic history can feel dangerous, psychologically speaking. It all goes back to the concept of stability. Uncovering secrets is a "big destabilizer," he says, especially when a family that thinks of itself as Christian finds out they might be Jewish. Grammy still doesn't believe we are Jewish. It's just too much for her to digest.

Nevertheless, Grammy is of Jewish descent. With her consent, our lab has used her genetic information (along with mine and that of other family members) to research BRCA1 mutations. Along the way, we've sequenced her whole genome, and her Ashkenazi heritage is clearly written into her DNA. Thanks to scientists who have sequenced the genomes of hundreds of Ashkenazi Jews, the Ashkenazi ancestry has been traced to about 350 people who lived around seven hundred years ago in the region that is now Israel. *Ashkenaz* in Hebrew means "Germany," and Ashkenazi Jews did indeed originate in eastern Europe and the Middle East. The genomes of Ashkenazi Jews are so similar that everybody in the population is a biologic relative to everyone else with a maximum of thirty degrees of separation.

I called Uncle Manny and surprised him: The mutation was inherited from Grammy's side of the family, not his. He was ecstatic. But since he was still Jewish and therefore had a higher risk of having one or more of the three founder BRCA mutations, he kept his appointment for genetic testing. He tested negative. The fact that Grammy carries the BRCA1 5382insC mutation and Uncle Manny was negative for all three Ashkenazi BRCA mutations means it's less likely, but still possible, that Uncle Jack, Aunt Evie, or even Grumpy also carried the BRCA1 5382insC mutation.

While the mystery of Jack's cancer still isn't solved, what's *really* mysterious is why for years I believed it was the key to the family medical history. All along, the secrets were buried in a place I hadn't thought to look.

How to Learn about Your Genetic Inheritance When You're Adopted

Andy, a colon cancer patient, has a cancer story that begins long before his cancer actually appeared. Andy was adopted in infancy. When he was grown and married, he, like many adoptees, wanted to learn more about his biological parents and their health history. He decided to locate his biological mother and father before starting his own family. He wasn't concerned about a cancer mutation; as a psychiatrist, he was more worried about mental disorders that have a hereditary component, like schizophrenia. Having children without knowing his hereditary risks, he felt, was irresponsible.

So, thirty years ago Andy signed up with an adoption disclosure registry. All registries and agencies are a bit different, but Andy's registry worked like this: If both the biological child and a parent register and are willing to meet, they are connected by the agency. However, if only one of the parties registers, this person has the option to do nothing until the other party registers or actively requests that the agency search for the missing relative. Andy's biological parents weren't registered, so he initiated a search. When the adoption agency finally found Andy's biological parents, Andy's biological mother agreed to exchange letters with Andy, but only with all identifying information removed.

They wrote letters for four years before she agreed to see Andy in person. They met in a coffee shop; he learned that his parents had been unmarried when he was born (no surprise) and that his father was a Catholic priest at the time (um, surprise). He asked about mental illnesses and other hereditary disorders like Huntington's disease. None, his bio mother assured him. But, she asked him, would he do her a favor? She and his father—who had left the church and had long been married to his mother—wanted Andy to remain a secret. No one could know that Andy was born while his dad was still a priest. What could Andy say? He agreed. They were all trying to keep the family system as stable as possible.

Andy and his wife, after a long wait, began a family and had two children. Then, at age forty-two, Andy was diagnosed with colon cancer. He contacted his bio mother to let her know.

"Well," she said, "you should know that there have been others."

Others? It would have been nice for her to have mentioned a history of colon cancer during their lunch. Who were these "others"? Brothers, sisters, cousins? His bio mother demurred.

Eventually, Andy was let out of the closet and allowed to have contact with his full biological family. And eventually, he found out that these "others" referred to not just "other people in our family with colon cancer" but "other children who had been born while your biological father was still a priest and whom we had also given up for adoption and kept a secret." In what must have been one of the most awkward family reunions on record, Andy and *all* the biological children attended a large family wedding in South Carolina. One of the "others" was about to cancel her regular colonoscopy (the delay or cancellation rate for colonoscopies is 50 percent) when she heard Andy talking about how he'd been successfully treated for colon cancer. She kept the date, and the gastroenterologist discovered tubular polyps, a precursor to colon cancer. The polyps were removed, and her life was saved.

Andy's case is extreme, but it's useful because this single story embodies almost all the challenges that adopted children can face when they're trying to track their genetic history. If you're adopted, here are some ways to get and give important information:

- Adoption disclosure registries work, so please register. Adoption reunion registries can be run by nonprofits, governments, or businesses, so registering with more than one is useful. It's especially wise to register well in advance of making family-planning decisions. Registering works because many past "closed" adoptions were closed by default—meaning that the biological parents may not have been asked whether they wanted open records (think *Philomena*). Furthermore, all states allow the adopted person access to non-identifying information about birth relatives. But the health information is incomplete, so it's still important to try to get in contact with your biological relatives (even if through an intermediary) for up-to-date health information.
- Ancestry.com is one of several useful genealogy websites that includes data from the U.S. Federal Census records from the

1700s through the mid-1900s as well as birth, marriage, death, military, and other records from the United States, Canada, South Africa, the United Kingdom, and European countries. You can send in a cheek swab and request that the staff look for markers that tell you about your heritage (African, European, etc.). If any of your biological family members have also sent in a swab, the staff can identify those relatives and put you in touch (with everyone's permission).

- It goes both ways. If you have a disease-causing mutation, do all you can to find and inform your biological family. If you don't know who they are, start by using the adoption registry or one of the online genealogy tools.

- If your biological family doesn't report a history of cancer, great. But if you developed cancer at an early age or have had an unusual type of cancer, summon the courage to seek genetic counseling. It's still possible that you have a mutation.

Sometimes adoptees believe that they carry an unusual burden—that unlike people raised by biological parents, they face a mystery about their medical heritage. It may help to know that this isn't true. Few people have a close-knit extended family that gets together for big, happy Thanksgiving celebrations and football games in the backyard. Few know the real and potential medical problems in their family. You have work to do, but you are not alone.

The Best Time to See Your Doctor

No matter who you are or how hard it has been to dig up your family's cancer history, there will come a time when you need to take the next step and consult with your doctor to ask about your risk of inherited cancer. It's always good to go into your doctor's appointment with as much family history as possible, but don't let a lack of knowledge be an excuse to put off a medical appointment indefinitely. Cancer doesn't wait for you to get your paperwork in order! The best time to see your doctor is when you've gathered as much information as you reasonably can, within a reasonable amount of time. Know that you can always return to your doctor if and when you learn more. As I'll explain later, it's very possible that your doctor will refer you to a genetic counselor, who will expect to receive updates from you as you learn more about your family's history—because almost no one gets a perfectly complete family history on the first try. In the next chapter, I'll help you navigate discussions with medical professionals. As with conversations with family members about cancer, discussions with medical professionals can be complicated by unclear speech and outright avoidance. None of us can afford to miss an inherited cancer syndrome because of poor communication. But, as you'll see, that's almost what happened to me.

Chapter Four

Is Your Doctor Truthy?
Are You?

IT WAS A SURPRISE to both Grammy and me that we had a BRCA1 mutation. But maybe it shouldn't have been. After I learned about my mutation and gave the news to Grammy, I thought a lot about that research study we'd all enrolled in, the one that was supposed to examine our family history for the possibility of cancer mutations and tell us if anything was found.

At first, it seemed to me that the researchers had dropped the ball. Not just that—they'd dropped the ball, let it roll into street, and watched as it slipped down a storm drain. They were supposed to tell us about our BRCA1 mutation, and they didn't. They had failed. But the more I thought about it, the more I realized that the situation wasn't so black-and-white. After all, Grammy had received that letter, the vague one that said, "We have some interesting information to share with you."

And then there was something I didn't like to examine too closely. Before I'd learned about my mutation, before I'd learned about Grammy's letter, I'd been in contact with the research folks myself. I had called once, just to check in to see whether there had been any new developments, and the counselor answered my inquiry cheerfully. "The cancers are clearly not hereditary," he said.

I was relieved. If the cancers weren't hereditary, my chance of getting cancer was no higher than that of the average person. But Sean, who was my fiancé at the time, was skeptical about whether I'd heard correctly.

"*Clearly not* hereditary?" he asked me. "Or *not clearly* hereditary?"

I brushed him off.

Now, as I tried to understand why it had taken me so long—ten years after Bea's death!—to get tested for a cancer mutation, I felt a bit shaken.

They'd tried to tell us, and we'd missed it.

We have some interesting information to share with you.

The cancers are not clearly hereditary.

I turned these words over in my mind. How could milquetoast phrases like this be deployed to carry such powerful news?

And how did we, in our cancer-prone, hyperalert family, fail to read between the lines?

The answer, as Stephen Colbert might have said on *The Colbert Report,* was that all of us—medical professionals, my mother, me—suffered from a case of truthiness. What's truthiness? In a 2006 interview for *New York Magazine,* Colbert (speaking as himself and not his character) explained that he coined the word to mean "something that seems like truth—the truth we want to exist." In my family's case, the experts were saying what was sort of true, but they said it in such an indirect way that it was hard to understand and easy to willfully misinterpret. My mother and I like to think of ourselves as brave enough to look behind truthiness and spot the actual truth, but somehow we just . . . didn't.

In the last chapter I talked about how to get straight information from your family about your cancer history. After you've re-searched your history, your next step is to take that family history to your doctor. Your doctor, in turn, might decide that you need a referral for genetic counseling and genetic testing. (I'll explain more about genetic counseling, testing, and risk management later in this book.) I'm a medical professional, and I know that most of us try our hardest to be straightforward, thorough, and helpful. But we're people, and cancer is a complicated, emotional topic for us, too. Sometimes we succumb to attacks of truthiness. And some-times our patients do things—like file away our letters or mishear our words—that make it hard for us to accurately communicate the truth. In this chapter, I'll help you spot the signs of medical truthi-ness, whether they're coming from you or your doctor, and suggest ways to drill down to the facts.

(Truthy) Things Doctors Say about Inherited Cancer

Sometimes doctors and other health professionals can unwittingly make inherited cancers harder to spot or prevent. Vague speech and poor communication are top reasons for this.

If you're reviewing your family's cancer history with a health pro-fessional, or talking about how a piece of medical information might affect you, it's a pretty safe bet that you all share a common goal: to get you good health care. You don't need to be suspicious or antago-nistic in these conversations. Nevertheless, it's smart to stay alert. When medical professionals won't look at you directly, they are more likely to tell it truthy rather than tell it like it is. Some words and phrases can signal that a doctor, nurse, or counselor is hedging:

- *Ummmmm* or *Well, actually* . . . Depending on the context, these phrases can signal that a doctor isn't comfortable with how the conversation is going. Listen carefully to the words that follow. Do you detect a whiff of truthiness?

- *I think . . . possibly . . .* Like a hedge of shrubs that obscures a backyard view, these words are often used to camouflage uncertainty. If a doctor doesn't know what's going to happen to a patient, it would be better to commit to that ignorance and say, "I don't know." Instead, many of us will hem, haw, and hedge.

- *The facts state . . .* Medical professionals love the facts. Facts are what make us professionals. But this phrase can be a sign that the doctor is standing a little too deep inside her comfort zone, afraid to help you understand what those facts mean for you.

- *It's proven . . .* Almost nothing in cancer genetics is proven. There may be good evidence to back up a doctor's assertions, but in medicine there is rarely *proof*. Evidence can point strongly to a particular outcome; proof is irrefutable. Doctors and scientists are trained to use both of these terms carefully. When I'm reviewing papers for publication in journals, the word "proof" sets off my B.S. detector. It's a word that almost always means that the science in the paper is sloppy. If you hear that *it's proven* that a person with your family background can't have a cancer mutation, or that *it's proven* that a particular mutation will always lead to cancer, or that *it's proven* that a particular genetics clinic and hospital delivers the best services, raise your eyebrows.

- *To be honest* or *At the end of the day* or *Here's the truth, straight from my gut . . .* These phrases protest too much. While they sound as if they're signaling honesty, often they're camouflage for a case of truthiness. They tend to mean "I'd rather not explain the incredibly cloudy reasoning that's brought me to the point I'm about to make."

Why is there so much truthiness in medicine? For one thing, doctors don't get a lot of professional training in communication, especially when the news might be difficult. Delivering complex information in a straightforward, understandable way is a hard task. And not all of us are born communicators. I try to be precise with my patients and to explain information in a sequence that makes sense to them, but it's a skill that I have to practice.

I'm always glad when a patient says, "Let me make sure I heard you accurately. You're saying that . . ." and then summarizes what I've said. It's a good opportunity to correct any mistakes. It also shines a spotlight on any murky language. Back when I was on the phone with that study's genetic counselor, I wish I had taken a few minutes to say, "OK, I want to be sure I heard you clearly: 'The cancers are clearly not hereditary.' It sounds as if you're saying that my family definitely doesn't have a known hereditary cancer syndrome. Is that right?" But I was so eager to hear some good news that I skipped this step. It would have been smart for me to prepare for the phone call by reminding myself that, deep down, I wanted accurate information. That even if I felt too scared to hear that I might have a mutation, I needed to know—not just for my own health but for the health of my family, as well.

Another reason doctors can be vague is that they might not know you well enough to anticipate how you'll react to a particular piece of medical news. I once had to tell two sisters that they were at risk for a family cancer syndrome. The first sister was shocked but calm, and she immediately agreed to both counseling and subsequent tests. The second responded a little differently.

"Oh, I've got the mutation," she said. "I know I do. Actually, I've already got cancer." This time, I was the one who was shocked. I asked how she knew.

"Because I've got cancer symptoms."

Her family history suggested that she was at risk for a syndrome that can lead to a half-dozen cancers. I asked her which kind of cancer she thought she had.

"*All* of them," she said confidently, and reeled off a list of symptoms: weight loss, excessive fatigue, night sweats, cold intolerance, decreased appetite, sinus pressure, hoarseness, occasional difficulty swallowing, possible ulcer, cough, chest burning, reflux symptoms, nausea, nocturnal urination, hot flashes, hip pain, shin pain, anxiety, stress, and insomnia.

Just to be safe, we considered each of her complaints carefully. Her physical exam and test results were normal—and in the end, her genetic test for a mutation was negative. And with the negative test, her symptoms resolved. Later, she admitted that when we first told her about the possibility that cancer ran in her family, she immediately spiraled down to her "bad place." Apparently, at the mere suggestion of a mutation, she'd imagined each and every symptom.

We doctors just don't know how patients will respond to information, and sometimes we feel a little burned by previous encounters that were emotionally heated. The result can be communication that is overcautious and timid.

Once I wondered if I had gone too far into timid territory. I had a patient who was so straightforward, so honest and quick-witted, that I nicknamed her "the Rocket." She tested positive for a BRCA2 mutation, so we contacted the Rocket's sister to come in for counseling and testing. The sister was completely unlike the Rocket. Despite having the beautiful-but-fierce look of a runway model, the sister's emotional state was fragile. She was terrified at the thought of testing and always seemed to have issues that interfered with having a test done: insurance issues, work issues, family issues. She was so tense that I found myself tiptoeing around her, as if she might explode—a situation that led me to privately think of her as "the Bomb." If I didn't keep talking to her about the BRCA2 test, she might not ever get it; if I talked about it too much, she might be scared off completely. When I spoke with the Bomb, I used lots of hemming and hawing language, like "reportedly," "maybe," "it's possible," and "I think . . ." I still don't know if this was the right approach to take. But this wasn't a case of doublespeak intended to cloud the truth. It was an attempt to speak in a way that she could understand.

If you suspect that a doctor is treading too lightly around a topic, offer reassurance that you are ready for the news. Some patients bark out, "Give it to me straight, Doc!" but that's such a cliché that it's hard to know if they really mean it. Some insist, "Tell me the worst-case scenario," but that's another tough request to honor. The worst-case scenario is, almost by definition, unlikely to happen. It probably doesn't accurately represent a patient's risk or situation.

Instead, use other means to signal your desire for truth. Bring in a pad of paper to take notes, or ask the health professionals if you can record the conversation. They'll always say yes. Have a list of questions ready. Look 'em in the eye. (If you look away for an extended time, they might think you're not quite ready for the conversation.) Bring a family member or a trusted friend as a surrogate pair of ears and eyes, or to voice tough questions. (Just don't bring in someone who will make you nervous or who will commandeer the appointment. We've seen spouses who won't stop talking long enough for the patient to get a word in.) If you have a friend who is a doctor, ask that friend to call your doctor's office and suggest, gently, that he or she will be looking over your doctor's shoulder. This is an effective way to encourage your doctor to work at the highest level possible. And don't forget to summarize the health professional's words and ask if you've heard correctly. All these steps show that even if you are feeling more like the Bomb than the Rocket, even if your voice shakes a little or you get emotional, you're still determined to hear the truth. You can even say, "I know I seem overwhelmed. It's true that I'm worried. But it's important for me to hear the facts in a way that I can understand."

Another cause of truthiness is time limitations. A doctor may have no more than twenty minutes with a patient, and there's only so much information that can be conveyed in the time available. Physicians don't usually have time to say everything that *could* be said, so they make on-the-spot decisions about what to say and what to cut out. Some doctors, especially those who work in overscheduled community clinics, are so busy seeing patients that they don't have time to delve into complex subjects like genetics. Sometimes they make things up. A recent case in point: A patient visited our clinic with a note from her doctor advising that, based on her family history, there was "little doubt that she has the BRCA1 gene." This patient had never had cancer and her family history of cancer was not strong enough for us to convince her insurance company that a test for BRCA1 or BRCA2 mutations was indicated. While it's true "she has the BRCA1 gene" (because everyone has a BRCA1 gene), statistically she probably doesn't have a BRCA1 mutation that would put her at a high risk for breast or ovarian cancer. If you sense that your doctor is rushed or perhaps a little out of his or her depth, it may be time to move on. You can always say, "Thank you; you've been really helpful. I'd like to understand my risk as completely as possible. Could you refer me to a genetics clinic?"

When a person's level of genetic risk is unclear, communication is even more difficult. And, unfortunately, a person's exact level of genetic risk is almost always unclear. In our clinic, when a patient is found to have a mutation, we give that patient a series of percentages that represent a full range of risks. There might be ten good but different studies that show a variety of possibilities, and sometimes a person's level of risk depends on how much cancer is already in the family. Take the PALB2 gene. Studies indicate that a person with a mutation in this gene has a 70 percent lifetime risk of breast cancer—but only when there's already a strong family history of cancer. If you've got the mutation but have a weak family history, your risk of getting breast cancer in your lifetime goes down to 30 percent. Although risk percentages are not always as straightforward as patients (or doctors!) might like them to be, almost anyone can understand them with the right explanation. (We'll talk more about risk statistics in chapter 6.)

In our genetics clinic, we try to describe the entire range of risk, because there is always uncertainty about what study might be the most accurate. Most families are small enough and their histories of cancer are imprecise enough that we are not confident that our risk estimates based on family history are accurate.

But not every medical professional shares the full range of variables. And almost unconsciously, some doctors cherry-pick the numbers and percentages they share with patients. Some tell patients only about the studies that suggest the least amount of risk. Others always describe the highest risk. A person with a mutation in the BRCA1 gene, for example, could hear:

Your risk of developing breast cancer is 87 percent; or
Your risk of developing breast cancer is 50 percent.

That's a big difference. Some doctors are simply more pessimistic than others. Other doctors, sensing that a patient needs some good news, will move to the optimistic end of the spectrum and park there for a while.

I suspect, though, that these differences in the presentation of information are not just about differences in physician temperament; they also may have to do with being too busy to follow the literature. How many doctors have time to read all the papers that might be published about this single narrow topic? Limit the playing field to doctors who also have time to talk to their patients about each of these papers, and you've got a small field, indeed.

Communication is complex. The best of us struggle to write and speak clearly; we all have times when we don't listen as well as we should. The system of medical communication needs a backup. That's why nurse practitioners, genetic counselors, and second opinions were invented. Like a detective trying to put together the clues in a case, you will find that sometimes the best way to get to the truth is to solicit multiple opinions, weigh their merits as best you can, and synthesize them.

If you think your doctor is being even a touch truthy, get a second opinion. You won't hurt your doctor's feelings. Doctors, like everyone else, are a little insecure; backup of any kind is welcome. When I first learned of my BRCA1 mutation and was deciding on the best way to reduce my risk, I think I called nearly every breast surgeon and oncologist in the country. And I frequently get calls from friends and family asking me to take a look at their sick friend's medical records and to call their friend's doctors to talk about their situation. This is something I love to do, and I think most health professionals feel the same way. We've got skills, and we enjoy using them to help our friends.

When Medical Records Lie

A few years ago I was applying for life insurance and had to answer the usual medical questions. I pulled out the medical record from my double mastectomy and bilateral oophorectomy (the prophylactic surgeries I had after learning about my BRCA1 mutation) at Brigham and Women's Hospital in Boston in 2004. *Diagnosis: breast cancer*, it read.

My first thought was, *Did I have breast cancer and they forgot to tell me?* Remember, I have an active imagination.

But then I brought myself back to reason. The whole point of the surgeries was that they were prophylactic. I'd had them in order to *avoid* cancer. As I put the pieces together, it seemed likely that the surgeon who had performed my reconstruction had entered the error while writing a hurried post-op note, and his error was copied from chart to chart as I went through the health system. Thankfully, one of my doctors went to an extensive effort to officially correct the record for me. It's a good idea to have a copy of your medical records in your possession; your doctor's office should provide this upon request. If you discover an error, ask your doctor to correct it for you—and follow up as often as you have to to make sure that it gets done.

There are also nefarious cases of patients gaming the health system for their own financial gain. Once, a patient asked us to keep his genetic mutation out of his medical record. He was dodgy about the reason, but eventually we learned that he was suing his employer, blaming the tap water at his workplace for his cancer. He knew that his mutation had caused the cancer, but he thought the lawsuit would bring a windfall to his wife. This lie meant that he had to keep his mutation secret from his children, who didn't know that they were at a high risk for cancer. Even the tolerant, easygoing Uncle Jack would have considered this brand of truthiness completely classless.

As my breast cancer "diagnosis" shows, the problem with medical misinformation is that it's hard to erase. Like a virus, an error or a lie will replicate itself in chart after chart, until it starts to look like truth. This is bad news for people who are reviewing their relatives' records and trying to understand their own health history. It means that it's always smart to cross-reference any medical records with your family's remembered history. You may not always know which is correct, but at least you won't make the mistake of thinking you know something that you don't really know. Record errors are even worse news for science. Errors in charts mean that scientists who are studying broad health patterns will base their conclusions on incorrect data. Without the facts, researchers may miss important connections or may make false ones that take years to unwind. Bad data gum up the works.

HIPAA: It Helps More Than It Hurts

When it comes to telling you the truth about inherited cancer, are U.S. doctors hamstrung by the Health Insurance Portability and Accountability Act? Maybe, but not nearly as often as you might think. Here's what HIPAA does and why it exists.

In 1994, a *Boston Globe* health columnist named Betsy Lehman was treated for breast cancer at Boston's Dana-Farber Cancer Institute. The Dana-Farber was then and still is staffed by the brightest, most caring physicians around. But at the time, the hospital—like most others—kept records, including doctors' orders, on paper. An oncology fellow wrote an incorrect order for Lehman's chemotherapy, causing Lehman to receive the wrong dose. No one in the health-care chain—the fellow, the attending physician, the nurse, the pharmacist, and so on—caught the mistake, and Lehman died. If Lehman had received her chemo across the street at Brigham and Women's Hospital, where electronic medical records for prescribing drugs were already in use, the software would have prevented the mistaken chemo dose. (Ironically, Brigham and Women's is where my own record got that "diagnosis: breast cancer" line. Electronic records reduce errors, but they don't completely prevent them.)

The Lehman case was the most publicized of a series of wake-up calls that happened around the country; other patients in different hospitals were also overdosed on chemotherapy because of errors in recording decimal points and because the usual systems of human checks and balances weren't working. A cry went up; it was clear that electronic medical records were needed. And with *that,* people wondered: When my health information is recorded digitally, who can access it? How can I protect it?

In 1996, Congress passed the Health Insurance Portability and Accountability Act, which orders organizations to protect their patients' health information from theft, loss, or destruction. The law was a direct outgrowth of the Lehman-like cases, the clear need for digital records, and subsequent fears that those records could be abused. It's been estimated that hundreds of people (nurses, technicians, clerks, doctors, therapists) see a patient's record in a single hospital stay. Prior to HIPAA, no laws governed who saw the record, what information they were able to see, and what they were allowed to do with that information.

It wasn't until 2003 that the HIPAA privacy rule became a reality. This delay was related to fears that the law would put doctors in a straitjacket. And at first, we all responded to HIPAA with extreme caution, worried that if we accidentally said the wrong thing in the wrong circumstances, we might end up in jail. Doctors and their staff stopped leaving voicemails; they removed office sign-in sheets; virtually no information was sent via snail mail. Then it became clear that this excess caution was not necessary, that the government was leaving doctors reasonable room to do their work and make their own judgment calls. In fact, in the first three years after HIPAA went into effect, there was only one criminal case brought against a health-care worker, a lab assistant who had the nerve to steal the identity of a dying cancer patient.

At the time HIPAA was passed, nobody predicted the positive power that would come by giving patients the right to say who had access to their health information. Since then, the quality of patient care has increased with the protection of our patients' information. With HIPAA has come data standardization and maintenance of patients' personal health information in a secure and confidential place.

Still, privacy is not always a good thing. The situation is somewhat like genetic testing; it's a never-ending process of assessment and improvement. There are examples of HIPAA getting in the way of important information. Usually this happens when a patient with a mutation doesn't want this status known by the rest of the family (who might also have the same mutation), and the doctor can't get in touch with the other members to let them know they're at risk. Sometimes HIPAA is frustrating when we want to check the medical records of family members but don't have the family member's written consent and getting that consent is logistically fraught (for example, when a family member is in the Peace Corps, is away at college, or just doesn't answer the phone).

More often, though, it's *fear* of HIPAA—or rather of lawsuits— that makes it hard for doctors to tell you what they know. Vague notification letters like the one Grammy received come to mind. A friend of mine once received a letter from her radiologist that was so vague and chipper, she assumed it was a solicitation for a patient satisfaction survey. She threw the letter out. Several weeks later, she discovered the letter's real purpose: to inform her of a questionable shadow on her mammogram and to have her book a follow-up test.

There's a lesson here for all of us. Whether they need to or not, health professionals have generally responded to HIPAA with fear. Now, when they need to reach you about something important, they might not feel that they're permitted to *say* it's important. They don't want to breach confidentiality. If you get a letter, text, email, or voicemail from an office, don't read a single thing into the tone of the message or the voice of the person. These messages are carefully crafted to avoid betraying information. You have to assume that the message is important, even urgent. Follow up. It might be nothing. (For example, my friend's second mammogram turned out to be fine.) But I wish that when Grammy had received her letter from the cancer study, she had said to someone, "I'm so upset about Grumpy's cancer right now that I can't deal with this letter. It looks like nothing, but can you read this over and tell me if I need to do anything?"

HIPAA really is good for patients most of the time. But arm yourself with the knowledge that it can lead to communications that are deliberately vague.

What about Me? What about You? How to Avoid Avoidance

I don't want to suggest that doctors issue indecipherable, sloppy pronouncements as their patients, poor things, sit helplessly in their chairs. Sometimes patients or families contribute to communications problems. An extreme example is the family of a woman with end-stage endometrial cancer. When one of our genetic counselors suggested there might be a genetic component to the cancer and the hospice physician confirmed this, the family fired the hospice workers and our clinic altogether. A day later, a hospice worker reported that a sign appeared in their yard. It read, "Trespassers will be shot!" Clearly, this family was not ready to talk—or think—about cancer or predisposing mutations.

Several years ago, a patient with breast cancer transferred her care to my clinic. My nurse and I noted that she'd been to several other oncologists. During our first interview it became clear that she probably drank too much alcohol. I brought up the fact that one of the most common environmental (that is, nongenetic) risk factors for breast cancer is alcohol. Her eyes started to shimmer. After the visit, she sent me a long email arguing that alcohol is *not* a risk factor and telling me that data on alcohol and breast cancer were "contaminated." I returned her email and attached research papers that demonstrate a link between alcohol and breast cancer. Within five minutes she replied, saying that my lack of sensitivity was too much for her and that she wanted another doctor. I was fired.

Months later, an email landed in my in-box. It was the patient again. She was in Alcoholics Anonymous and wanted to return to our clinic for follow-up. As of this writing, she's been sober for many years and is cancer-free.

Similarly, when some people learn that they carry a cancer mutation, they minimize the results, as in the case of a woman who recently came to our clinic with thyroid cancer. She knew that she carried a mutation in the RET gene that can predispose to thyroid and other cancers. But for years she pretended that the mutation wasn't really all that significant. She could have taken steps to prevent cancer, but she missed the opportunity. Others bury the results of genetic testing entirely and pretend they've never had a test. When we see situations like this at the clinic, it's tempting to ask ourselves, How can someone be so neglectful? In reality, the psychology of self-deception allows us to filter out the things we don't want to hear or think we don't need to hear. In the phenomenon known as Morton's demon, we see only the evidence that fits with our current theories. I'm not immune. If I transposed the words of the phrase "not clearly hereditary" to "clearly not hereditary," it was Morton's demon that made me do it.

We all seek internal consistency. Psychologists use the term "cognitive dissonance" to describe the pain we feel when new information (for example, you learn you may have a genetic mutation) conflicts with an existing status (you don't see yourself as a person with a genetic mutation). Denial is one way we attempt to avoid the pain of dissonance. Facts can be scary and, for a little while, ignorance can be bliss.

Of course, denial works because we don't recognize it as denial. At the time, denial seems like something else—like common sense, or sound thinking, or being thoughtful of another person's feelings. It's much easier to recognize denial when it's coming out of someone else's mouth. Here are some statements people make when they're desperately trying to reduce cognitive dissonance:

> *I can't possibly need genetic counseling. It's obvious that the cause of my cancer is my agony over the divorce.*
> *I can't come in for a test. I'm too busy at work.*
> *I live too far away to get that blood test.*
> *You doctors just want to use me for research.*
> *God will heal me, so there's no need for testing.*
> *Lots of people in my family died from cancer, but all those cancers have nongenetic explanations. My brother and mother died from stomach cancer because they were mean. I don't need counseling.*
> *This test result says I have a mutation, but the lab technician probably made a mistake.*

Do any of these sound familiar? If so, don't waste time being hard on yourself. You're in excellent company. Just recognize that although denial brings a soothing sense of internal consistency, that comforting feeling doesn't last for long. The pain of cognitive dissonance will return eventually. If you're feeling a bit truthy even as you read this book, try talking to a friend or a health professional. When you express your denial out loud to a caring person, you might find that the denial loses its power. You can also imagine your life ten years down the road. Thinking about your hopes for the future can pierce your current denial.

Knowing that genetics gives you options you didn't have before is another powerful but positive way to reduce dissonance. If the young woman with the RET mutation had understood that risk-management decisions could have reduced her cancer risk by 90 percent, she might have taken action and prevented her thyroid cancer. Learning about a cancer mutation isn't about hearing bad news that we'd be happier not knowing. It's about taking control and making choices before our bodies make them for us.

In the case of one patient who believed that prayer would heal her case of inherited cancer, we stepped in to explain that she could pray *and* have medical care at the same time. Then we switched to providing an external piece of information: "If you take care of yourself, you will help your family." This is often a persuasive argument that works even with a serious case of denial, and even when families are estranged. Let me say it again, but this time I'm saying it to you directly:

If you take care of yourself, you will help your family.

Repeat this as often as you need to. And say it to family members who need to hear it. Without this kind of firm statement, many people will be too overwhelmed that their genetic reality doesn't meet their expectations. They'll stay in denial—in the way that Grammy continued to believe that Bea died of breast cancer because she was "too stressed."

Cognitive dissonance is a tricky beast. Even if *you've* accepted a medical truth about yourself, you might see denial at work in other people, as they seek to explain their own bewildering feelings about your health. When the actress Angelina Jolie publicly announced that she had a BRCA1 mutation and had decided to undergo prophylactic mastectomies, people felt anxious—even those people without a family history of cancer. To justify this anxiety, they engaged in their own form of denial, which unfortunately can look a lot like criticism or blaming. That's why, in the days after Jolie's announcement, you heard people "explaining" why she didn't really need the surgery or suggesting that she was going to lead a trend in unnecessary procedures. These were people who weren't ready to accept that Jolie had made intelligent, powerful decisions that probably saved her life. It's particularly hard when people close to you do not accept the existence of whatever situation you're in. You may feel pressure to change your views so that they conform to everyone else's—even when everyone else is wrong. Don't give in. Reassure yourself with a combination of data, expert opinion, and your clearest thinking.

Ultimately, the best cure for denial is to know that we're all capable of it. And to remind ourselves that things that sound good should never win out over good, sound reasoning. Holding on to our comfortable opinion today will make tomorrow much more uncomfortable. One of my colleagues was recently diagnosed with colon cancer at age sixty. He told me that he regretted not having had a colonoscopy at fifty. To quote him: "There is no better way to learn than passing through your comfort zone. I sure wish I'd taken on the discomfort of a colonoscopy ten years ago rather than taking on chemotherapy now." People who refuse to see that they're at a high risk for cancer are missing one of the twenty-first century's greatest opportunities.

Chapter Five

Genetic Counseling, Genetic Testing, and Family Conversations

IF YOUR DOCTOR HAS SUGGESTED THAT you might be at risk for an inherited cancer syndrome, or if your family history shows any of the signs that cancer might be in your genes, the next steps are meeting with a genetic counselor and (maybe) getting genetic testing. Genetic counselors aren't just kind people hired off the street; these folks have master of science degrees in genetic counseling; in the United States, they must be certified by the American Board of Genetic Counseling. They blend a deep knowledge of genetics, genetic conditions, and risk management with the ability to support people who are learning information that could feel overwhelming. Your doctor can refer you to a genetic counselor. You shouldn't have to travel very far, because many hospitals have a genetic counseling center. You can also find a list of certified counselors on the National Society of Genetic Counselors website, nsgc.org.

If you take a look at many genetic counseling pamphlets and websites, you'll see a lot of pastel colors, pictures of roses, and beautiful people gazing thoughtfully through windows. The implication? Genetic counseling and testing are like days at a spa, with professionals who talk softly and tread lightly. But this is not true. Patients cancel their visits to the genetic counselor as frequently as they do their colonoscopies. It's stressful.

The stress, of course, comes from wondering if you'll find out that you're at increased risk for cancer. Even more stressful should be not knowing whether you're at risk. Or wondering if you're *not* taking advantage of actions that can save your life. Whether to get genetic counseling is a personal decision. My ultimate, but delayed, choice to get genetic counseling was an easy decision. The delay was more about denial, not about counseling. In this chapter, I'll walk you through the process of genetic counseling and testing to make it easy for you, too.

Do You Need Genetic Counseling?

It may be hypocritical of me to urge you to get genetic counseling, because I spent at least a decade putting off my own counseling appointment. In the years after Bea died, I tried telling myself that my family's pedigree—the one I'd drawn by hand after her death—didn't reveal any patterns that might indicate inherited cancer. I also told myself that it was useless to investigate my family cancer history much further. Why should I bother, I asked myself, when the conversations would be so hard? I kept my mind off my own genetic history by staying deeply involved with my twin missions of caring for cancer patients and doing basic cancer research.

Then I was diagnosed with melanoma. Both Sean and I knew that when a dark-skinned, sun-avoiding person gets melanoma in her thirties, it's smart to check for a cancer mutation. Sean pressed me to get counseling and testing. Still, I wavered. The reason I stayed away from genetic counseling went deeper than grief or being busy or hesitant to have awkward conversations with my family. I can admit now that I felt scared. I was scared of having an increased risk of cancer, but I was also scared that if I learned I had a genetic defect, the people who loved me would leave me.

Sean and I were newly married, and we were in the process of weaving together a new family with two children from his previous marriage. My dad had recently died, and we were helping my mom, Grammy, acclimate to life as a widow. Although my melanoma had been easy to treat, we were still recovering from the shock of the diagnosis. On top of everything else, it was almost Christmas, and everyone was burdened with the usual strains of the season. If I carried a genetic mutation for cancer, would my new marriage reach a tipping point—and tip right over into separation? Divorce?

Against this backdrop of fears that I would be unplugged from my new family, I remembered something hopeful. I thought about what Bea Wiz said about hard situations: that the goal in life isn't to avoid difficulty; it's to be comfortable with our own imperfections and the imperfections of others. Once, when I was around eight years old, Uncle Manny's kids were visiting us at our Michigan lake house, which we all called "the cottage." The children's room was a big, open loft at the top of the cottage, and one day the cousins and I were up in the loft when we got into an argument. I can't remember what we were fighting about, but even though it was probably something inane, our bickering turned into yelling. Suddenly, we heard a book slam down, hard, on a table in the family room. We realized that Bea had heard us. We went silent and peered over the side of the loft in fear. Bea was sixteen years old, fiercely loyal to us, and hardly ever angry. So when we realized we'd made her mad, we knew we were in big trouble. Bea was heading toward the screen door to leave the house, but she turned and stared up at us.

"I'm disgusted!" she said. "We have a great life here. We're so lucky to have each other! And you kids can't see that. Instead, you're wasting the day fighting over something stupid!" Then she walked out.

Her reprimand stung. We stopped arguing and began to play cooperatively.

After a while, Bea returned and came up to the loft. She explained that she was glad we'd stopped fighting—but that even if we hadn't stopped, she would have understood. "You can't help it," she said, "because you're not yet fully formed people."

That was Bea in a nutshell. She was still a teenager, and she could sound a little supercilious, but her apology was real. Even as a teenager, she instinctively understood that the only way to really connect with people is to meet them where they are and to love them as they are (fully formed or not). And that's all any of us has to go on. I loved Sean and my families, both old and new, and I'd give them a chance to accept me, possible mutation and all. I took a deep breath and, as a holiday gift to myself, I emailed Charis Eng, M.D., Ph.D., the leader of the Clinical Cancer Genetics Program at the Ohio State University and booked an appointment to meet with Eng and her genetic counselor (Heather) on a day in early January.

Talk to a bunch of genetic counseling patients and you might start to wonder if you're at an Alcoholics Anonymous meeting—because over and over again, you'll hear people describe how it took them a long time to see the light and how they hit rock bottom (in the form of a health crisis, like my melanoma) before getting the help they needed. As the saying goes, if you're asking yourself whether you're an alcoholic, you already have the answer: You are. If you're asking yourself whether you should get genetic counseling, you should. It's that simple. Your doctor can write you a referral.

Here are other indicators that it's time to see a genetic counselor:

* Your family's pedigree shows a pattern of inherited cancers. You can learn more about how to spot inherited cancer syndromes starting on page 27, and you can also consult appendix 1.

- Your family's pedigree doesn't show a clear pattern of inherited cancers (mine didn't), but you still have questions. Read pages 35–38 for help creating your family's pedigree.
- You frequently worry about whether you carry a genetic mutation for a particular inherited cancer syndrome.
- Your doctor suggests you get a genetic assessment.
- Your friends or family members are telling you to get a genetic assessment.

Despite my nervousness about making the appointment, I was unexpectedly content when the day of the appointment arrived. I had a whole day to spend with my hubby—no clinic, lab, kids, or other duties to worry about. I nostalgically recall the four-hour drive on wintry roads from Ann Arbor, Michigan, to Columbus, Ohio. I read stories from the *New York Times* aloud while Sean drove. When we tired of that, we alternated between listening to Bach (my choice) and AC/DC (Sean's). We drove past snowy cornfields under a gray sky, watching the landscape stretch out for miles ahead of us. Near Columbus, we stopped at a Panera. It was so cold outside, and the restaurant was invitingly warm. Sean and I relaxed over chicken noodle soup, and I enjoyed the feeling that on this trip we were members of a team working together for the sake of good health, seamlessly coordinating our efforts. Every time I visit a Panera, I think of that trip, order some soup, and feel warm.

How Genetic Counselors Can Help You

A genetic counselor will walk you purposefully through the details of your family's particular patterns and risks and decide whether to recommend genetic testing. If testing is recommended, your counselor will see you through the process, help you determine the level of risk, and support you through the next steps. He or she will even help you contact other family members if it appears they're at risk.

Going into my appointment, I knew all these things about genetic counselors. But I was surprised to learn that my genetic counselor would know a lot about my health-insurance company and what it would and would not pay for. Genetic counselors also know what the insurance company will pay when it comes to health-management activities brought on by the results of your genetic analysis, whether it's close surveillance with frequent doctor visits, scans, blood tests, and colonoscopies, or it's prophylactic surgeries such as colectomies, thyroidectomies, or mastectomies. Don't underestimate the value of this benefit of counseling! Genetic testing is getting cheaper all the time, but it still costs real money to have tests performed by a reputable lab. Insurance companies can and will deny claims for tests that are inappropriate. Let's say that you have a family history of cancer and that breast cancer in particular is on your mind and emotionally wrenching because your aunt had it. You ask your gynecologist to test you for BRCA1 and BRCA2 mutations. The insurance company denies your request for preapproval and you feel outraged. How could an insurance company deny your right to know if you're at risk for cancer? You want the tests, so you agree to pay out of pocket. The results come back; you don't have a mutation. You finally get to a genetic counselor to help you understand your negative test results, and you find out that, given the specifics of your family history, the counselor would have predicted the negative test result. You also find out that because you mainly have a family history of thyroid cancers, you qualify to be tested for a mutation in a different gene: PTEN. Patients with PTEN mutations are at risk for thyroid cancer, and—less often—colon and breast cancers. You're stuck with the bill for that first test—and you still need to have the correct test performed. A counselor will find out whether your health insurance covers genetic testing and, in collaboration with the laboratory that will be performing the test, help with the preauthorization process. (Some labs can manage the preauthorization process themselves, but a number of good but small labs don't have the bandwidth to deal with insurance companies and effectively handle preauthorization.)

Genetic counselors also know which testing labs are the best. In 2013, the U.S. Supreme Court ruled that BRCA1 and BRCA2 (and any other genes, for that matter) cannot be patented. Since then, tests for genes and their mutations have been proliferating like fruit flies; so are quacks who are trying to make a quick dollar and take advantage of the overburdened regulatory programs that oversee for-profit labs. Ms. Carter, a patient of ours, visited her doctor, located in a small Texas town, because her sister had been found to carry a BRCA1 mutation. The overworked doctor recalled that a representative from a genetic testing company had left a sample testing kit and some pamphlets around the office. But instead of testing Ms. Carter for the specific mutation that her sister had, the testing company—let's call it WTH Labs—analyzed the entire sequence of both her BRCA1 and BRCA2 genes and reported to the doctor that Ms. Carter did not have a mutation in either gene. The patient was reassured and told to celebrate. She and her children had been handed the lucky straw.

But then Ms. Carter developed breast cancer. Her doctor began to question the test result and sent Ms. Carter to us. Our genetic counselor smelled a rat. Why would the lab test for *all* the possible mutations of both genes, rather than just testing for the specific mutation that was already known to run in her family? Genetic tests are expensive, and it's poor practice to test for more than the mutation already known to be in a family. And the specifics of the lab result weren't available. Why not? We called the lab, and it refused to recognize that there was a problem. We then sent Ms. Carter's blood sample to a different lab, one we trusted, for retesting. Ms. Carter did indeed have the same mutation her sister had. The first lab had blown it. Fortunately, Ms. Carter's cancer was still treatable. And fortunately, both genetic counselors and clinical geneticists are trained to ferret out disreputable labs and to make sure you're working with the good guys.

Even more important, a genetic counselor can spot patterns of cancer that may be moving through the family. Your counselor will create his or her own pedigree of your family; it will help if you've drawn your own pedigree and filled it out as completely and accurately as possible. Then the counselor will look for signs that could point to inherited cancer syndromes: multiple cases of cancer (two or more close family members on the same side of the family with the same or a related cancer); a person who had cancer at an early age; or a person who has had more than one kind of cancer. And then there are certain types of cancers that are so rare that when they occur, counselors always suspect the presence of an inherited cancer syndrome, even if only one member of the family has had that cancer. These include ovarian cancers, male breast cancer, and adrenal gland tumors. Of course, if it's already known that your family has a mutation, then the counselor will make sure that you're checked for that specific mutation.

Another reason to see a genetic counselor is that a counselor will help you face the genetic truth, even if you'd prefer not to. Self-deception is real. I'm a doctor and a scientist, but as I sat in the chair opposite Heather and Dr. Eng, I was certain that our meeting was an exercise in excess caution. I was sure that I wouldn't need a genetic test. When both Heather and Dr. Eng recommended that I get tested for a BRCA1 and a BRCA2 mutation, I agreed, thinking that I was humoring them. When Sean and I stood in my Michigan office, listening as Heather told us that the results were in—that I had not only a mutation but also a particularly aggressive one—I realized that these genetic experts had saved my life. Without their supportive but firm insistence, I would not have undergone the test.

Denial aside, genetics is *hard*. A master's degree in genetic counseling requires about two years of course work, research, and clinical instruction, plus additional continuing education. In contrast, many doctors haven't studied genetics long enough to make an accurate assessment of a pedigree and to know the best next step. It's not that they're bad doctors. It's just that genetics is a complicated specialty that takes time to learn. I lean on our clinic's certified genetic counselors, led by our alpha counselor Linda Robinson, every day with every patient. This expertise is the primary reason that the National Comprehensive Cancer Network (a consortium of cancer experts in the United States that suggests standard of care guidelines in oncology) recommends counseling before genetic testing.

Heather had called me before our initial meeting to take a family history, and when I sat down with her and Dr. Eng, I was delighted to find that she'd already drawn a fresh new pedigree for me. She emphasized the importance of obtaining medical records, when possible, to confirm cancer diagnoses in affected relatives, and she was game for trying to get the elusive records for Aunt Evie and Uncle Jack. We arranged to have release forms sent to the hospitals, and she said she'd let me know if we received confirmation of the diagnoses.

Heather and Dr. Eng agreed with the assessment I'd made long ago: There was no clear pattern of inherited cancer in my family. *See, I was right all along!* I wanted to crow. However, they also said that there was enough cancer to warrant searching for a possible mutation. I felt a little less like crowing then. But which mutation should I be tested for? Because my father was Jewish, and most of the cancers were on his side, they decided it was logical to begin by looking at my risk for the Ashkenazi Jewish mutations in BRCA1 or BRCA2. To determine my risk of having a mutation, Heather and Dr. Eng used resources that I didn't have, including statistical models and laboratory data that take into account personal and family history as well as ancestry. Testing is considered appropriate for anyone with more than a 10 percent chance of having a mutation; the models placed my risk for a BRCA1 or BRCA2 mutation between 29 and 37 percent. They took my blood for testing and also, I was glad to see, for research.

Genetic counselors are better than palm readers at predicting the future; they are, in fact, skilled at interpreting future cancer risk. They also reflect the human side of the science. Heather was not only sensitive to how stressful test results can be but also clear in telling it like it is. She was, and remains, available to answer questions for her patients.

But even a great genetic counselor can't pull all the weight in a counseling session. You'll get much more out of it if you take an active, not a passive, role in the discussion.

Get the Most from Your Genetic Counseling Appointment

Most genetic counseling appointments last around an hour. To get the most out of that time, arrive prepared. Draw or create your family's pedigree online before the appointment (like me, you may first have a phone appointment that's dedicated to discussing your family history) and bring a copy with you; be clear about where you have accurate information and where you're not sure of the truth. Remember that making up information or guessing can mislead your counselor and send both of you stumbling a long way down the wrong path. If you have medical records, family medical histories, or other written information, consider bringing them along for reference.

Sometimes patients walk into our clinic and say, "I know I need a genetic assessment, and I want to take responsibility for my health. How do I do that?" We love it when this happens. The first thing we do is tell these patients to gather a family history as best as they can. Another way I answer this question is to describe an ideal patient who has a strong family history of cancer. Ideal patients are committed to their health and to the health of others. They undergo testing when it's recommended, without making excuses or putting it off. If they're asked to participate in genetic research, they eagerly agree. If they find that they have a mutation, they do not feel or act like victims. They're simply glad they've found what is wrong with them, and they begin to research their options (more on this subject in the next chapter). Ideal patients see the value of getting help and staffing up. They have small egos; they are not narcissistic. They realize they may have blind spots, so they talk with experts to get clarity. These wonderful, superpowered people also understand that, as the complexity of genetics increases, the need to rely on genetic counselors increases.

Best of all, these ideal patients don't care what the world will think if they have a mutation. This is a reason I'm a fan of people like Angelina Jolie and Christina Applegate. After being diagnosed with breast cancer at age thirty-six, Applegate was found to have a BRCA1 mutation. She chose to have a prophylactic double mastectomy to avoid future cancers. She also formed a very successful nonprofit that cancer geneticists respectfully call the "Applegate Fund" (officially it's Right Action for Women). This charity pays for breast MRIs for underserved patients that are at a high genetic risk for breast cancer. These funds are a godsend for our clinics, as we see a large number of underinsured patients from the two safety-net hospitals associated with UT Southwestern Medical Center (Parkland and John Peter Smith Hospitals). Even with the Affordable Care Act, the copays for these patients can be too high, and Applegate's charity steps in to foot the bill.

Jolie's and Applegate's choices to disclose their BRCA1 mutations, to have surgery, to share their experiences as a way of helping others, and to do all this with elegance and simplicity are admirable. Before Applegate and Jolie, both Betty Ford and Gilda Radner helped make cancer less secret and more matter-of-fact. To people like Applegate and Jolie, there is no such thing as genetic helplessness.

It may go without saying that I was not one of these ideal patients. It wasn't just that I was in denial. There was a moment when I flashed back to my less-than-stellar years in grade school; sitting in the genetic counseling office, I felt like I was being called out by my fourth-grade teacher, Quick Jaw McGraw, for yet another infraction of the code. Mrs. McGraw stood at the front of the room and spoke so fast it was similar to having bullets whiz by your ears. Hence the nickname. One solution was to cuff the ears with the hands. As an alternative, one could focus on the prize, the playground, which was easily viewed through the back window. This was considered inattentive. This time, though, I wasn't just failing to pay attention or simplifying taking a standardized test by filling in the same answer in each row, all the way down. I felt like I was failing—period. I felt embarrassed and even ashamed. How I could be in denial while also feeling guilty is a matter for psychologists to sort out, but in my work at our genetics clinic I see that I'm not alone in trying to manage these conflicting feelings. If you're not an ideal patient, you have plenty of company. We get through the best we can. Still, it's helpful to have role models like Applegate and Jolie, to know that there are others who've been through testing and who've approached it as a job that needed to get done. Know that it's OK to feel confused and upset and worried. But when you do, think of these role models and say to yourself, *Genetic counseling is a job that needs to get done. That's how I'm going to approach this.* You might find that if you act the part, you grow into the role. And then you can become a model for the people who come after you.

What Happens during Genetic Testing

After your blood is drawn, it's shipped via FedEx or another company to a testing lab. At the lab, the white blood cells are burst open and your DNA is separated from proteins and other molecules. Although it's often said that your DNA exists in every cell of your body, that's not quite true. Red blood cells, for example, don't contain DNA. Blood itself can be tested for cancer gene mutations because of the DNA contained in your white blood cells.

After lab workers isolate your DNA, they use sonic waves or enzymes to cut it into fragments. Then the fragments of DNA are copied using a process called polymerase chain reaction, which increases the amount of DNA that the lab can work with, making their job much easier. Next, these millions of copies go into the sequencer, a piece of equipment that looks like a fancy refrigerator. Remember that DNA is made up of four nucleotides, or bases: A, T, C, and G. These four letters (or bases or nucleotides) write the blueprints for your cells; what those instructions say depends on the order in which they appear. DNA sequencing is the process that allows us to read the letters in the order they appear in your genes (if individual genes are sequenced) or entire chromosomes (if your entire genome is sequenced). In my case, the technology used old-time Sanger sequencing, named after the two-time Nobel laureate Frederick Sanger, and only the nucleotides within my BRCA1 and BRCA2 genes were sequenced. But 2004 was several years ago. Now labs use more advanced sequencing technologies that allow them to sequence several genes at the same time, and to sequence them faster. This process is known as next-generation sequencing.

Next-generation sequencing has dramatically reduced the cost of sequencing. The first genome took ten years to sequence and cost three billion dollars; today, powerful computers routinely reassemble all the information from the millions of DNA fragments from a single genome into a coherent sequence within a few days. This increase in speed and drop in price is due to lots of market competition and disruptive technologies across several fields, including microscopy, surface chemistry, nucleotide biochemistry, computation, and data storage. DNA sequencing has advanced in ways that were inconceivable when I had my test done. (Nevertheless, it's still much less expensive to sequence one or a few genes with technical accuracy than an entire genome. More important: Even though we have the technology to sequence whole genomes, we don't understand 99 percent of the sequenced material. That's why you get screened for only the mutations you're at risk for.)

More than 99 percent of the nucleotides (those building blocks of DNA) in each person's genes fall in the same predictable order as everyone else's. The few genetic differences among individuals tend to be the ones that encode the differences in our inherited traits—from the color of our eyes to our cancer predisposition. To locate the differences in your gene or genes, scientists compare the sequence of your genome to that of a reference genome. Think of the reference genome as a normal gene sequence shared by many people. It's like the template composite genome of an average human. Nobody actually has a completely "normal" genome. Some of your abnormalities can reduce your cancer risk, while others can increase it. Most have nothing to do with cancer at all. Every face has both flaws and beautifully unique characteristics; so does every gene sequence.

Our lab recently sequenced a number of patients from the clinic using a reference genome known as genome research consortium human 37 (GRCh37), which is derived from thirteen anonymous volunteers from Buffalo, New York. These volunteers had been screened by genetic counselors, who eliminated those with an obvious genetic syndrome, before donating their blood for DNA analysis. The human reference genome is stored in GenBank, a site managed by the National Center for Biotechnology Information, and among reference genomes, it's considered to be a strong, reliable one. If your sequence varies from the reference genome that the lab is using, it's checked against other databases of sequence variations to determine what kind of variant you have and what that variant might mean for your health.

What about Direct-to-Consumer Genetic Tests?

Why meet with a genetic counselor? Why can't you do all this work on your own by using a mail-order genetic test? These direct-to-consumer tests (known as DTC tests, for short) allow you to bypass the medical profession altogether. The DTC company will mail you a testing kit. At home, you collect a DNA sample (usually a cheek swab) and mail it back. The company then contacts you with the test results. By law, DTC genetic testing companies can tell you only which mutations they have found. They can't tell you what most of those mutations mean. And that's the biggest hitch in the DTC process. As I'll explain later in this chapter, we *all* have genetic mutations. It takes an expert to understand which mutations are potentially harmful, which are benign, and which fall into the frustrating category of "significance unknown." If you get a DTC genetic test, you'll need to see a genetic counselor to understand the results. And even then, most genetic counselors prefer to work with the labs they know and trust—so know that a counselor could toss out the DTC test and order a new one.

Understanding the Results of a Genetic Test

Since the results from any genetic testing can be a challenge to interpret, your counselor or doctor will work to educate you about the findings. But sometimes what they are saying can sound like the teachers speaking in a *Peanuts* episode: *Wah wa-wah wa-wah wah wah waaaaah wah wa wah. . . .* So here's a simple framework on which you can hang your results. There are three main categories of results:

- *yes,*
- *no,* and
- *maybe.*

Yes

Yes means that you've tested positive for a mutation that increases your risk for cancer. The lab test calls such mutations "deleterious" or "pathogenic." You inherited this mutation from one of your parents, *even if neither of your parents has had cancer.* This result has consequences for your family. If you have siblings, each one has a fifty-fifty chance of inheriting the mutation; if you have biological children, each one also has a fifty-fifty chance of having inherited the mutation from you. Your extended relatives could have the mutation as well. If you are the first in your family to learn that you have a mutation, you get to be the leader (even if in real life you are a follower) and help the rest of the family get tested.

Your genetic counselor should tell you exactly which gene is mutated. Your counselor will also tell you the specific nucleotides that are "misspelled" in that gene. In my case, the BRCA1 gene is mutated, and the specific "misspelling" is BRCA1 5382insC. Remember, everyone has the BRCA1 gene; when it's fully functioning, this gene protects against breast, ovarian, and other cancers. When the BRCA1 gene develops certain mutations, they alter the structure of the protein and prevent it from doing its job. Some of the mutations are thought to be more deleterious than others. This is true of other inherited cancer syndromes as well. There's almost always a range of risks. Each range represents varying results of different studies. It also represents the way that the risks vary according to your family history. Someone with my particular BRCA1 mutation and my strong family history of cancer is, generally speaking, on the higher end of the risk of developing breast or ovarian cancer. Someone with the same BRCA1 mutation but no family history may fall in the lower end of that range. (For more information about the range of risks associated with some inherited cancer syndromes, see the chart in appendix 2.)

A yes result does not mean that you will definitely get cancer. It means only that you are at an elevated risk. For me, that risk is high. For someone with a different BRCA1 mutation and no family history, the risk is more moderate. For every mutation that I've listed in this book, you can take positive steps to manage the risk. For some, those steps involve prophylactic surgeries or medications; for others, it's increased screenings. In the next chapter, I'll talk more about strategies for managing risk—and managing your worries.

No

No means that you don't have the mutation for which you were tested. If you were tested for a specific mutation because one of your family members has tested positive for it, you have a very clear result: You don't have that mutation. In all likelihood, you are done with testing.

But if you have a strong family history of cancer and no other relative has been tested yet, it's possible that you still have a mutation other than the specific one that was tested for in that gene or in another gene altogether. For example, I was tested for the panel of common Ashkenazi Jewish BRCA1 and BRCA2 mutations. My test came back positive for the BRCA1 5382insC Ashkenazi mutation, and we had an explanation for many of our family cancers. We have the hereditary breast cancer and ovarian cancer syndrome. But if the test had come back negative, Heather would have recommended looking for other mutations throughout the entire sequences of the BRCA1 and BRCA2 genes. If those also came back negative, then—as she explained in our initial counseling session—we still wouldn't be done. My family had several cancers that were not tightly associated with BRCA1 or BRCA2 mutations. Those included Jack's supposed adrenal cortical cancer; Grumpy's adrenal cancer (pheochromocytoma) and melanoma; and my own melanoma—all of which could possibly suggest different genetic syndromes. If I tested negative, the next tests in line would be for Li-Fraumeni syndrome (a mutation in the tumor-suppressor protein TP53) and familial malignant melanoma syndrome (caused by, for example, a mutation in the CDK2NA gene, also known as p16INK4a). Because of Grumpy's pheochromocytoma, I may also have been tested for Von Hippel–Lindau syndrome (VHL) and multiple endocrine neoplasia type 2 syndrome (MEN2). My family history certainly didn't loudly declare a specific syndrome. But it did suggest that an inherited mutation or two could be there and that it would be smart to analyze more than a few genes before concluding I carried no known mutations and our family cancers were just a boatload of bad luck.

If lots of people in your family have had cancer and they test negative for several mutations, it could be that your family members share a common nongenetic risk factor, like exposure to carcinogens. It could also be coincidence. But of course, not all mutations are known yet. We're discovering new ones all the time. If you get a series of *no* results, you may need to return for testing when new cancer genes are discovered or when you learn something new and significant about your family history. A 2014 study showed that women with a mutation in the PALB2 gene who also had a significant family history of breast cancer were at a higher than previously known risk for breast cancer—up to six times the risk of the average person. This discovery explained why some women with a strong family history of breast cancer had tested negative for mutations to the BRCA1 and BRCA2 genes. If you test *no* for a mutation but have a family history of cancer, stay up on the medical news and in touch with your genetic counselor in case there are new tests for you. Genetic analysis and testing isn't a onetime event; it's an ongoing health habit, like getting your cholesterol checked or going to the dentist (and certainly more interesting). In the future, a yearly checkup with a geneticist to update your family history and testing status could become the standard of care for everyone.

Maybe

Maybe means that you have a variant of uncertain significance. We don't know what these variants mean in terms of your cancer risk. As more and more people are tested, we are gathering more information about these indeterminate results and what they mean. Eventually, variants of unknown significance will be reclassified as either harmful or, more likely, harmless.

To put things in perspective, everyone has genetic mutations— *many* genetic mutations. On average, each of us has 815 variants of unknown significance scattered throughout the coding regions of our estimated nineteen thousand genes. (The coding region, which encodes proteins, consists of just a small percentage of the entire genome and is where we find most cancer-causing mutations. It's currently not possible to estimate the number of variants found in noncoding regions.) Researchers at times call these coding region mutations "potentially pathogenic variants," but don't let the phrase scare you. The potential for problems here is very low.

Some variants of unknown significance are called "loss of function" mutations. In these variants, the gene is not able to make a complete protein or makes a protein that is seriously defective. Each of us, on average, carries ten of these broken genes. Mind you, most are not harmful, either because the gene is not necessary for health or because you have a backup copy of the gene that can do all the work on its own. Remember that you have two copies of each gene: one from your mother and one from your father. For some genes, one good copy is enough. For other genes, the acquisition of additional defects in some of your cells in the good copy of the gene (called "somatic" mutations, because you don't inherit them in all your cells but rather acquire them in only certain cells as a result of bad luck or exposure to mutagens like cigarette smoke, alcohol, or UV radiation from intense sunlight) can lead to disease. BRCA1 is one such gene. People who are at increased risk of cancer as a result of inheriting mutations in one copy of BRCA1 from one parent typically acquire mutations in the other copy of BRCA1 in certain breast or ovarian cells. These cells lack any functional BRCA1 protein and consequently lose their ability to maintain the integrity of the rest of their genome. They go on to develop additional mutations in cancer genes, ultimately transforming those cells into cancer.

Some patients and doctors prefer not to think of variations in the genome that are likely deleterious as "mutations"—instead they use the word "variations" or "changes." But I've come to like the word "mutations." It feels like a badge of honor. It feels real.

A variation in a genome can be essentially meaningless. It's as if a word in your genetic code has been misspelled but in a way that doesn't alter its meaning. Sean spells his name S-e-a-n, but sometimes people will spell it S-h-a-w-n. Sean understands that both spellings refer to him, and he responds to them both. If you have a *maybe* result, it could be caused by one of these insignificant misspellings.

Even large variations in a gene may not lead to any problems. You can be missing a big chunk of a gene and still not have an increased risk of cancer or any other disease or disorder. It's similar to someone calling you by your first and last names but forgetting your middle name—usually, it's no big deal. You still know that you're being called; you still function the way you're supposed to.

Getting the News

Learning your test results is a big event, and your reaction is bound to surprise you. One of the counselors at our clinic talked to a man whose brother had died at a young age from colon cancer due to a Lynch syndrome mutation. When she delivered the news that the man was free of the mutation, he sobbed—vigorously and at length. At first she was concerned about him, but later he happily explained that he was relieved and that this had been his first really good cry in thirty years.

There is no single "correct" response to learning your test results, whatever they are. My own reaction to learning that I had a BRCA mutation was shockingly upbeat. After all those years of denial and suppressed worry, I felt purposeful and energized. I finally had an explanation for the cancers that plagued my family and now could not only take steps to manage my risks but also help others in the family manage their risks. I would have never guessed that I would have felt this way, and of course not everyone does. It's normal to feel fear (what if I get cancer or already have it?); anxiety for your children and other relatives (what if they have the mutation, too?); guilt (I should have gotten tested sooner!); shame (am I defective?); surprise (how could this happen to me?); grateful (to past patients who participated in research); and glad (I finally have an answer and a plan). Some people who have never been sure they wanted to have biological children feel a mix of relief and guilt, because a mutation gives them a concrete reason not to. Negative results can also elicit puzzling emotions, from relief to freedom, guilt, or even frustration that you don't have a clear explanation for family cancers. This tangle of emotions is just one more reason to work with a genetic counselor. If you send your blood or cheek swab off to a lab yourself, or if your doctor does it for you without genetic counseling, you'll miss the benefit of having the results delivered by a person trained to help you through your response.

There are four things to remember as you prepare to hear your test result. First, it's never easy to face life-changing news, especially when you're buried in a long list of daily to-dos. However, a test result may lay wonderful waste to the perceived importance of those daily chores. When I found out I had a mutation, I was in the middle of writing grants, supervising postdocs and grad students, seeing patients, and caring for our children. Getting the news reassembled my priorities. I knew that I wanted to have prophylactic surgeries, but I also wanted to investigate my options for those surgeries. I put off the grant writing, stopped micromanaging the postdocs, and hired my most child-friendly graduate student to do some extra babysitting.

Then I made a new list of things to do, and I did them systematically. I made sure to spend focused, non-distracted time with the kids. I talked to surgeons and oncologists, studied the research about prophylactic surgeries, made sure my insurance was in good standing, kept my extended family informed, and finally scheduled surgeries at my hospital of choice (Brigham and Women's Hospital in Boston). It was all interesting and engrossing.

But again, not everyone responds this way to the news of a cancer mutation. After Bea's daughter reached adulthood, she was tested for the family's mutation. When she learned she tested positive for the BRCA1 mutation, I asked her, all aunty with solicitude and caring, if she was OK.

"It was terrible!" she said.

I began to reassure her that the positive result was going to give her options and choices. No matter what her decision, her mother would be proud of her bravery for facing the truth.

"No, no," she corrected. "I've always assumed I was positive for the mutation. But I just hated getting my blood drawn for the test. That was the terrible part. I almost fainted." As it turned out, Bea's daughter had accepted the reality of the BRCA1 mutation long ago. She'd already integrated it into her identity.

My patient Masera from Michigan had yet another reaction altogether. When she discovered a mutation that predisposed her to all kinds of cancers, she decided to pour her daily vodka down the sink and start restoring old cars, a dream activity that she'd never gotten around to. Masera is still sober and free of cancer, and she has lots of award-winning restored cars.

The second thing to remember is that genetic tests look for mutations in known cancer genes. As mentioned above, there may be other, currently undiscovered mutations that could affect your cancer risk.

Third, testing positive for a mutation doesn't mean that you will get cancer—and testing negative doesn't guarantee that you will never get it. Try to avoid a fatalistic mind-set.

The fourth and final thing to remember is that unless you are in the middle of a cancer diagnosis already, you don't have to make any decisions right away. You have time to think about your next steps. Your genetic counselor is there to help you understand your mutation and what you can do to acknowledge its existence and manage your risk. (The next chapter will help you to make decisions that are best for you.)

We Need "Mystery Patients" to Help Us Understand the Genome

If you're a "mystery patient," one with a family history that indicates a genetic predisposition to cancer but with no known mutation that can be identified with current genetic tests, then you'll need to stay in close contact with your genetic counselor. If a new test is created, your counselor should let you know about it—but don't sit back in your recliner and wait to be notified. Call the clinic every year or so to ask if there are any new tests you should have. Again, don't rely on your family physician or ob-gyn to know about the current tests. You need to stay in touch with the genetic experts.

I also urge mystery patients to participate in research. The only way for science to identify new mutations and develop new tests is to have genetic material available for study. The human genome has an estimated nineteen thousand genes. We have useful information for about four thousand of them. We have some idea about what it means when each of these four thousand genes is broken. But the full function of each gene—why it prevents disease, and how to use genetic information to prevent disease—is still a steaming pot of mysteries. Researchers can now readily sequence a patient's DNA, but our genetic code is written in a language that science doesn't understand very well yet. We recognize the alphabet, but in most cases we don't know how to read the words.

Science knows the human genome about as well as I know Spanish. I know just enough to have a five-second conversation with Oscar, the Spanish-speaking man who picks up the trash in my office at night. Every evening, I say, *"Hola, cómo estás?"* He says, *"Bien."* Then I say, *"Hasta mañana"*—unless it's Friday, in which case I say, *"Feliz fin de semana."* Either way, he yells, *"Adiós!"* and slams the door. The rest of Spanish is unknown to me. That's what our current understanding of the human genome is like. And there is no Rosetta Stone or Berlitz program to help us learn the language of the genome. There's no comprehensive translation dictionary to help us look up human genes and their meanings. We're not always sure how to tell the difference between a standard spelling and an alternate spelling—or a serious misspelling, representing a variant that can cause diseases like cancer. Massive amounts of research still need to be done to complete the first version of the genome dictionary.

In my laboratory, we are working with other labs to connect each nucleotide to patients and their families' cancer predisposition. By doing this, we hope to identify more genes that are like BRCA1, BRCA2, MLH1, and APC. These are all genes that, when intact, get the job done. They keep the cell's DNA and protein factories neat and tidy, and they keep cancer at bay. When you inherit one broken copy of one of these genes, your risk of cancer increases because the second copy can be broken by somatic mutations in certain cells of your body. If researchers keep sequencing more genomes of people with cancer in the family, we'll find more of these genes, and we'll learn more about what happens when these genes are mutated. Eventually, we'll be able to help more people understand and manage their genetic risk for cancer and other diseases.

Effects on Your Insurance Policies and Employment

If your genetic test uncovers a deleterious mutation, a federal law called the Genetic Information Nondiscrimination Act (GINA) will protect you against some forms of discrimination. For example, GINA makes it illegal for your health insurance provider to require you to disclose your genetic test results, or to make its decisions about your coverage and eligibility based on those results. The law also forbids employers with more than fifteen employees from making hiring, firing, and promotion decisions based on genetic tests.

There are some loopholes. GINA doesn't apply to businesses with fewer than fifteen employees. If you're in the U.S. armed services, or if you receive benefits from either the Department of Veterans Affairs or the Indian Health Service, GINA doesn't apply to you. The law also doesn't extend to life, disability, or long-term care insurance.

It's possible that insurance companies will soon catch on to the value of genetic knowledge. If you have a genetic assessment, test positive for a mutation, and then follow the guidelines for prevention and screening, you might be deemed a bargain to the company. Someday, perhaps there will be higher costs for those who *don't* have genetic analyses, in the same way that insurance is more expensive for those who smoke cigarettes.

Telling Your Family about a Mutation in a Cancer Gene

When you get your test results, those results don't stop with you; they affect your blood relatives. Your genetic counselor will help you figure out who is at the most risk and which members of your family should be contacted first. But if you test positive for a cancer mutation, it's ultimately your job to tell every blood relative you can find. The most important aspect of this communication is giving your relatives accurate health information and an idea of next steps. This may feel daunting for you. It can feel like a burden that's piled onto your shoulders at a particularly hard time. But you are giving your relatives a gift of potentially lifesaving importance. You would want them to tell you if you were at risk.

Who's going to tell your family members that they may have inherited a cancer mutation? The job usually falls to the first person who tests positive. In my family, that person was me. This was a new role for me; I was used to thinking of myself as the youngest child, the one who always hoped to be as good as the elders and tried to follow dutifully but never quite seemed to have the same level of responsibility. Maybe that's why my first call didn't go as smoothly as it might have. Remember that Heather and I had initially identified my father's family as the most likely source of the mutation because of their cancer histories and because it made sense. I had a Jewish mutation and they were Jews. Heather pinpointed my father's brother, Uncle Manny, as the person who was the most at risk. We agreed that I would call him and explain that he should be tested for the same BRCA1 mutation. As I've mentioned before, I called to give him the news. What I didn't mention is that I was completely unprepared when Manny began to cry. Now, Manny has a history of crying for all of us. When Bea died, he lost liters of tears. At Grumpy's funeral, Manny sobbed through his eulogy. Crying is not out of character for him. This time, though, Manny was crying because he has five children, four of whom were women in their late thirties and early forties at the time—and as a psychiatrist and man of medicine, he knew that this age is the prime time for problems from the BRCA1 mutation to surface. One of these daughters was pregnant. If I had taken a few moments to put myself in Manny's place before I made the phone call, I might have been less surprised at his response.

I delivered the news to most of my family by phone, but therapist Carolyn Daitch suggests that email may be a good choice, too. An email, she points out, might seem less personal, but it gives people a chance to absorb and reflect on the news. You can attach health information from your counselor or doctor that your family member can either read on the spot or tuck away for a moment when they are ready.

What if you need to tell someone who isn't likely to be receptive to your news? You might have to deliver your message to a relative who is estranged, difficult, or tends to avoid hard topics. In these cases, therapist Jerome Price recommends a strategy he calls "successful and benevolent" manipulation: Send an email, but don't give away all the information. Instead, write a teaser in the subject line, something like, "You have a fifty-fifty chance of carrying a genetic mutation for cancer. Please email me back for more information." Even if the person isn't likely to open a message from you, she or he can't avoid seeing the subject line. If you don't hear back from the person in two weeks, follow up with another message that delivers the full information.

Should you ever let someone else deliver the news? In touchy situations, look for an "in"—a family member who has the most credibility with everyone else or who is usually responsible for communicating important information. This is often a parent or an older sibling. Or, in cases of extreme estrangement, follow Price's suggestion to take advantage of family anxiety and let it work for you. Look for the person who is going to be the most concerned, even scared, by the news. That person will be the most motivated to listen to you and to take action. Tell that person, and then ask him or her to work with you to tell the rest of the family.

The confirmation of a cancer mutation is like a boulder tossed into the family pond. It's a big enough deal that it can create ripples of fear—but it can also disrupt old, dysfunctional patterns. In the way that funerals can become a time when people let go of their hang-ups and reconnect, talking about a mutation can lead to good change and family togetherness. This good change might not happen all at once, so have patience. Give your family members information. Then wait. Give the system time to assimilate the news. Keep dropping information so that the news can't get pushed underground. If the family still doesn't respond, consider seeing a family therapist, who can help you figure out ways to get information to your family members.

Genetic test results can challenge how families understand themselves. Hidden pregnancies, paternities, adoptions, or births that involve surrogates or sperm donors can be revealed. A patient came in to see me for testing because she'd been diagnosed with two melanomas before the age of twenty and then a breast cancer in her thirties. Her mother came with her for the appointment and sat through the family history intake. When the test results came back, the patient learned she had a CDKN2A mutation. When a single copy of this gene is mutated, it causes a syndrome that increases the risk of melanoma. (This is one of the genes that Heather had told me they would've investigated in my family if my BRCA1 and BRCA2 tests had come back normal.) My patient's father had died, so we couldn't test him for the mutation, but I informed the mother that she should come in for a test, in case the mutation was passed down through her. Later, the mother called me to explain that no test was necessary. Her daughter was adopted and didn't know it. I suggested the mother tell her daughter about the adoption and then work to inform her biological relatives of the mutation. Her daughter could also ask for important health history information from these relatives. This was one of those boulders in the pond, a chance for the mother and daughter to reorganize their relationship.

Genetic tests can also bring fears and old hurts to the surface. One of our patients, Joe, is a son, a brother, and an uncle, but his biological family bonds are weak. Because of his father's alcoholism, he sought "family" elsewhere—with friends and colleagues. Then Joe was diagnosed with stomach cancer and found out he had a CDH1 mutation. When it's normal, the CDH1 gene makes a protein, E-cadherin, which helps neighboring cells stick together to form tissues; the protein also prevents out-of-control cell growth. When CDH1 is mutated, a person has a higher risk of hereditary diffuse gastric cancer and lobular breast cancer.

Since Joe had a CHD1 mutation, some of his biological relatives almost certainly had it, too. Despite this huge risk to his relatives, Joe was hesitant to let his biological family know. He worried that the news would trigger his father's drinking and that the family would be angry and accusatory. So Joe rationalized that his poor diet made him more susceptible to stomach cancer than the rest of the family and that no one else needed to know. Eventually, he emailed a form "family letter" to his relatives. For him, that was the most contact he could bear. His willingness to find a way to communicate showed that he understood the information's life-sparing potential.

How families communicate depends on how they see themselves. Is the family a haven from the storms of the outside world? A business? A sports team? Some themes, whether spoken or unspoken, are "we are responsible for those less fortunate," "you can always do better," "seize the moment," and "you can always depend on family." That last one was our family's theme. When I realized this, I finally understood why Grammy initially didn't want to tell anyone she had breast cancer and why Bea wanted to keep her metastatic disease to herself. They thought that they would no longer be the ones that their family could depend on.

Ethnic heritage is also important. In some cultures, families have a "privacy boundary" so that family members feel secure in knowing that what they tell relatives won't be shared with people outside the family. In cultures that don't encourage open communication, emotional turmoil can be expressed in physical pain, including stomach problems or headaches. Jewish families are more likely to discuss everything ad nauseam. In the Jewish community there is a high level of family-related motivation to be tested for colon and breast cancer genes, in the hopes that the knowledge will help future generations. But these are loose generalizations, and all families are different. In one family with a history of cancer, a woman may independently make the decision to get tested, whereas in another family, all medical decisions may rest with the husband or a dominant grandmother. It's important to know what your family's patterns are. Then you choose to work with them—or to break from them if necessary.

Chapter Six

How to Manage Your Cancer Risk When Information Is Limited

IF YOU'VE GOT A MUTATION THAT predisposes you to cancer, you can take real action to lower your risk. This wasn't always the case. In the old days—and by "old days" I mean the early 1990s—if you had a family history of cancer, all you could do was sit around and wonder if and when you'd get it. Things are different now. Screenings and prophylactic surgeries can save your life. Still, there might not be medical agreement about the best way to reduce your risk. This chapter is about how to make decisions about managing your risk, even when the experts give you conflicting information, or when you don't have all the data you'd like.

I often compare myself to a detective, and I tell people who are tracking down their genetic inheritance to think of themselves as detectives, too. I tell them to gather the facts and follow the trails, even when the trails seem cold. But if you are making decisions about managing your cancer risk, I want you to stop using this comparison and shift to another. If you think of yourself as a detective, you can get stuck in Sherlock Holmes mode—believing that if you could only be more observant, gather more information, and process everything you know in just the right way, you'll land on the one correct answer.

But let me say this now: You're never going to have complete information, because that's the nature of medical decisions. You have to make the best decision you can with the information you've got. This means that, at some point, you're no longer a detective. You become more like the president of a country. You've got a situation you need to resolve. You've got some data, but not as much as you'd like. You've got some advisers, but some of them disagree. In this chapter, I'll explain the recommendations for common inherited cancer syndromes and how to make decisions that help you manage your cancer risk.

Cancer Risk Management and the Powers It Brings

I can't say this often enough: Despite what other people tell you, there are no black-and-white decisions when it comes to risk management. There will always be judgment calls. For a patient with the mutation for familial adenomatous polyposis, the lifetime risk for colon cancer is nearly 100 percent. The only known way to prevent an early death from colon cancer is to have the colon removed. This is a case when surgery is clearly effective and necessary. But even here, there can be variables to consider: choosing among capable surgeons, the timing of the surgery, etc.

Most decisions involve even more difficult judgments, because most mutations don't carry a 100 percent lifetime risk of cancer. Your risk might be more like 50 percent, or 80 percent, or 30 percent. Who gets to say when it's "right" to have a preventative surgery or when it's "wiser" to take more conservative measures, such as undergoing screenings or adopting healthier habits? Neither decision is objectively better than the other. The right decision for you depends on many variables beyond your risk of cancer. How treatable is the cancer or cancers you're at risk for? Can it be caught early through screenings and then treated successfully? What would that treatment look like? What are the consequences of prophylactic surgery? How anxious are you about the possibility of getting cancer? How anxious are you about surgery? These decisions reflect who you are, where you are in your life, your values, and the nature of your support systems. These decisions are a great opportunity for you to show your best side.

People may tell you that making decisions is easy. First, you figure out what you'll gain or lose from each decision; then you choose the one that leads to the most gain. Those kinds of decisions really *are* easy. But what do you do when the gains and losses are not clear? What do you do when your lists of pros and cons come out equal? What do you do when both options seem good? When both seem bad?

Making decisions that are not black and white is like learning a new subject. Everybody learns at their own pace and in their own way. If you try to force the process, or if you try to learn the way somebody else wants you to, you learn less. I don't learn in groups. I need to be in a quiet space with no interruptions. Others learn *only* in groups. Listen to yourself. Know yourself. You might be facing choices that feel immense, complicated, and life changing—but you probably also have some experience making complex decisions. You've had to decide where to live or where to send your children to school or whether it's worth working for a bad boss in order to advance your career. So draw on your experience with making complex decisions.

Think about your ideal conditions for making choices. Maybe you need time alone to weigh your options. Maybe you need to hash things out with several different people. Maybe you need to think for a few months, then stop thinking, and then think again. I make decisions through a process that looks like procrastination. From the outside, it seems as if I'm dillydallying. I practice my golf swing. I doodle. I meditate. I consider taking yoga classes. On the inside, though, I'm internalizing each different scenario, trying them on to see how they fit. It's like bringing a collection of clothing into the fitting room; it takes me a while to try them all on. When I'm ready, I model a few in front of the sales agents and ask for their input. This decision-making strategy may drive the people around me nuts, but I have to mull things over on my own timetable. And it's not just the decision-making process that's personal. The decisions themselves also have to be right for you. If you choose not to have a prophylactic surgery that's recommended by the experts, like an oophorectomy to reduce your risk of ovarian cancer, you're not doing anything illegal. It's *your* choice. No one can force you. Your responsibility is to listen well, to get the facts, and then to make a choice that is sensible for you. Making conscious decisions that acknowledge the facts gives you power.

Risk Management Options for Common Family Cancer Syndromes

There's a four-step process to cancer risk management:

1. Know whatever information is available about your risk.
2. Know your options for limiting that risk.
3. With the help of counselors, doctors, friends, and family, select among the risk-management options that are the best fit for you.
4. Act.

The first two are somewhat straightforward. A list of common inherited cancer syndromes can be found in appendix 1, along with, in appendix 2, their typical risks of cancer and the currently recommended options for limiting that risk.

The options for risk management vary with inherited cancer syndromes, and the recommendations for some syndromes can be very precise. In general, the options tend to fall into four broad categories.

First, there are lifestyle changes. Almost all experts agree that stopping smoking, moderating your alcohol intake, exercising, and using sunscreen can be helpful in reducing cancer risk. I simply stopped drinking alcohol when I knew I had a high risk for cancer (plus Grammy's father was an alcoholic, and I wondered if there might be a genetic tendency toward drinking too much). I also take a jog—some might call it Prancercise—around my neighborhood each morning. There is evidence to support additional lifestyle changes if you are at risk for certain cancers. For example, people at risk for colon cancer should moderate their consumption of red meat. These lifestyle changes involve almost no risk and can boost your overall health. Still, if you have a high genetic risk for cancer, lifestyle changes are rarely enough.

Another management strategy is increased surveillance. This can include yearly colonoscopies, frequent imaging of breasts with MRIs and mammograms, biochemical tests of blood and urine, or other screenings, depending on the cancers you're at risk for. These are all low-risk, relatively noninvasive options. The downside is that screenings don't prevent cancer; they just try to catch it early. Sometimes screenings fail to spot cancers. A false negative can mean false reassurance.

In some cases, medications can effectively decrease your risk. Birth control pills can help prevent ovarian cancer, aspirin can help prevent colon cancer, and tamoxifen can prevent breast cancer in some women.

But no drug can prevent cancer to the extent that prophylactic surgeries do. Prophylactic surgeries remove the tissue(s) at risk, such as breasts, ovaries, fallopian tubes, uterus, thyroid, stomach, or colon. Surgeries can be the most effective way to reduce your risk. Of course, prophylactic surgery has lifelong consequences, and it can be a tough choice for some people.

This chapter will not serve as a full risk-benefit analysis of each of these options. I list them here simply to help orient you before going into the decision-making strategies below.

Difficulties in Decision Making

Making medical decisions is so hard for some patients that doctors have a name for the problem: decisional paralysis. I don't love that term. It suggests that something must be wrong if you don't choose among your options right away. The reality is that you've got a right to wrestle with your choices and to take your time making them. Still, it's helpful to know that there are some predictable difficulties in making risk-management decisions and that there are ways to cut through them. These difficulties include the following:

- Confronting loss,
- Facing medical uncertainty,
- Sorting through conflicting information,
- Choosing among equal options, and
- Managing external pressures.

Confronting Loss

Prophylactic surgery is the removal of an organ that is prone to cancer. If you're contemplating prophylactic surgery, you are considering a physical loss, and that can be hard. When I opted for mastectomies and oophorectomies, I lost both of my breasts and my ovaries. There were other losses, too. Ovaries regulate estrogen levels, so I went into an immediate menopause. I naturally "run hot," so I always imagined that I'd have an easy adjustment to hot flashes when the time came. Instead, I was surprised by the intensity of my hot flashes. I also experienced some irritability and fatigue. Although I can't be 100 percent sure of the reason I felt this way, I was happy to pin both problems on the oophorectomies, which can make it harder for the body to modulate itself. I had to have patience as I waited for my energy and normal mood to return.

I was also surprised at what I gained. I opted for reconstructive surgery and was delighted with the results. I think I lost a few pounds, too. Possibly the weight loss was in my imagination, but what the heck—sometimes a vivid imagination comes in handy. And when I was in the throes of the surgeries, I didn't feel obligated to answer emails immediately. It also occurred to me that having preventative surgeries was nothing compared with what happens when a soldier loses a limb or a person dies of cancer, so I didn't feel too sorry for myself.

That said, I often found myself griping about the fact that medicine isn't simple, clear-cut, and unambiguous. Why was it so hard to make decisions about which surgeries to have? True, it was easy for me to decide on mastectomies and oophorectomies once I learned that I had a mutation. It probably looked as if I'd made an instant decision, but I'd been fretting about my risk of breast cancer for so long that I had slowly, and not completely consciously, worked up to it.

But I also had another surgery to think about: removal of the uterus. The association between BRCA1 mutations and endometrial cancer is weak, but when you have a family history of endometrial cancer, the risk is slightly higher than normal. And I did have a family history: Grammy had endometrial cancer in addition to her breast cancer. And it is possible that Aunt Evie's mysterious "ovarian" cancer was actually endometrial cancer. In this case, I didn't know what I wanted to do. So, on days like this, days when I was irritated and undecided, I'd call my friend Janet. She'd commiserate for a while, but eventually she'd say something useful, like "Just move on, dear. We all need you to get some work done." Janet was right. Take a look at anyone who is really living his or her life, and you'll see a person who is making tough decisions right and left. I was lucky to have a friend who could kindly point this out.

It's natural to worry about how your looks will change after prophylactic surgeries, especially mastectomies. I was worried, too. Then I realized I was thinking too much about the standards of beauty set by glossy magazines. Forget those! What, I wondered, were *my* standards? How do *I* like people to look? I thought about what I appreciated in the looks of my colleagues and friends. I don't like to be surrounded by disheveled, dirty, drooling people. I like to work and play with people who are clean and twinkly-eyed. It's fine by me if they *aren't* all strikingly beautiful. In fact, I prefer it. If we were all gorgeous, we'd get nothing done, outside of staring at one another, luxuriating in our beauty. I found this attitude—that I want to look like the kind of person I want to be friends with—tremendously helpful. I decided that I wanted reconstructive surgery, but I didn't want to turn the process into a total makeover. In other words, I went for the Dolly Parton personality but not her physicality, if you know what I mean.

I understand that there are others who think differently. I had one client who seized the chance to get the biggest fake boobs *ever*, and she's delighted with them. Some people say, *If I'm going to be under anesthesia, I might as well get my eyes lifted, too.* And there are magical and artistic plastic surgeons who can remove fat from your belly and place it in your breasts. Prophylactic surgeries involve loss, and we all process that loss in our own ways. My observation is that the people who land on the other side most successfully are the ones who balance the loss with a physical or psychic gain.

Coming to terms with the loss of an organ is easier when your family history already has you scared. By the time our patients with the familial adenomatous polyposis mutation—the one that carries close to a 100 percent risk for colon cancer unless the colon is removed—learn that they have it, they've already seen several family members die at a young age. It's clear to them that with the surgery, they are gaining decades of life. As another example, hereditary diffuse gastric cancer syndrome carries such a high risk for stomach cancer that people who come to our office often *hope* we discover a mutation in the family, because it means that those without the mutation are no longer at risk and those with the mutation can get their stomachs removed and know that they can avoid the fate of their siblings, parents, and other relatives.

It's harder when the mutation comes as an out-of-the-blue surprise. One of our lovely patients, whom I'll call Ms. Adora, was recommended for genetic counseling because she developed the rare cancer pheochromocytoma (the same cancer Grumpy had at age fifty) when she was only twenty-seven years old. Everyone has two adrenal glands, and she had the one with the tumor removed. We tested Ms. Adora for mutations in several genes and hoped for the best—that we'd find out her cancer was just a fluke, or that the pheochromocytoma was caused by a mutation that was unlikely to do further harm. That didn't happen. It turned out that Ms. Adora has the RET mutation, which not only leads to rare adrenal cancers like pheochromocytoma but also comes with a 95 percent lifetime risk for medullary thyroid cancer.

Ms. Adora was shocked. She notified her family, and everyone who tested positive for the same mutation will follow the guidelines and have their thyroids removed. In addition to thyroid removal, Ms. Adora and all her family members with the RET mutation will need to be followed for pheochromocytomas, with yearly urinary tests of metanephrines, metabolites of adrenaline that are produced by pheochromocytomas. They will also need to be tested yearly for calcium levels in their blood to screen for tumors of the parathyroid gland. To make things harder, Ms. Adora and her husband have a one-year-old son. We usually don't test children for genetic mutations, because most mutations don't pose an elevated risk for cancer in childhood. Instead, we wait until they are eighteen. But some RET mutations are exceptions to this general rule, and the mutation that Ms. Adora carries can lead to thyroid cancer in children. If Ms. Adora's son tests positive for the mutation, he will need to have his thyroid removed by the time he's five years old. At his age, his risk for pheochromocytoma is low and we would wait until age eighteen to test his urine for metanephrines. It's a lot of information for a parent to handle, especially since the mutation came as a surprise.

There is good news for Ms. Adora, however. The thyroid produces thyroid hormones, which control your body's metabolism. Without enough thyroid hormone, you become tired and cold; with too much, you become jumpy, hot, and bothered. After her total thyroidectomy, Ms. Adora can take a thyroid replacement hormone medication that will almost completely manage her symptoms. Most thyroidectomy patients are surprised to find that with the medication they feel as good as they did before the surgery, except that they get hot faster when exercising and cold sooner when resting. That's because the thyroid medication keeps hormone blood levels constant, whereas an active thyroid gland is constantly regulating those levels in response to the environment. Although there are some patients who don't have a smooth ride and experience fatigue, weight gain, depression, and other side effects, the vast majority of people (95 percent) who are on thyroid hormone replacement therapy have only minor side effects, or none at all. Those who do have problems can sometimes find relief by switching to one of the natural freeze-dried drugs (porcine, bovine, or a mixture of both) that are made from animal thyroids. Having a thyroidectomy is still a loss, but Ms. Adora is ready to accept it.

Some people face loss by temporizing. One of our BRCA1 patients is almost thirty-five years old and at a high risk for breast and ovarian cancer. She's not ready for surgeries; recently engaged, she hopes to have children soon. Yet she wants to do something to modify her risk. We suggested that she start taking the drug tamoxifen, which can help prevent breast cancer in women we predict are at a higher risk. The tamoxifen could affect her fertility, so even this nonsurgical alternative carries a risk. However, she knows she can stop taking it at any time. It's a compromise, but she thinks it's a good one. She plans to further reduce her risk with surgeries when she's older.

But there are losses that are less tangible, such as security, family, or friends. I actually felt closer to my family and friends after I learned about my mutation; it became a project that we could work on together. But I worried about my career. Even though I worked as an oncologist as well as a scientist, I was afraid that if people found out I had a BRCA1 mutation, they would see me as fragile and wouldn't consider me for interesting work. When it came time to inform my immediate boss that I would need time off for preventive surgeries, I wrote him an email explaining my situation. (I used email so that he would have time to mull over the information and pull together a thoughtful response.) He wrote back, quickly, to say that he needed the exact dates of my absences and that I should fill out some paperwork. That was it. No "That's big news. I'll be thinking of you." Or even "Maybe this is an experience you can use in your work with oncology patients." Later I realized he was busy with many more immediate issues and my story was one of many employee stories that he'd heard over the course of a week. Still, I was transiently irritated, and when I told Sean about it, he felt the same. At that point, we decided that since we couldn't assume a helpful response, we needed to limit the discussion of the matter among our colleagues. (Sean's lab was also in the cancer center, so the staff in our two labs interacted quite a bit.) First, we pulled together a message that he told his team. It went like this:

> You may have noticed that I've been unusually busy and stressed lately, and I thought it important to share with you some personal information, as I may continue to have less time available, and I may seem distracted at times in our meetings over the next several months.
>
> Some of you may already know that Theo was diagnosed with melanoma in the fall. She had surgery, we caught it early, and all indications are that she is cured. However, as a result of this, and the very strong history of cancer in Theo's family, we recently sought genetic counseling. We have been advised that there is a high probability that Theo could develop certain additional cancers. As a result, we have been spending a lot of time over the past few weeks meeting with doctors and surgeons to discuss ways of prophylactically reducing Theo's cancer risk. Theo has not been diagnosed with any new cancers, her life is not in danger, and we expect to be able to resolve all these issues over the next several months. However, the medical issues are complex and distressing. As a result, Theo and I are quite preoccupied as we work to resolve them.
>
> I am sure that you can understand that this is personal and know that you will respect our privacy by keeping this information confidential. I realize that you may be concerned, but please don't ask for updates or additional information from me or Theo as we're still trying to figure this stuff out ourselves.

I used similar language in a message to my own colleagues. I was glad that I had clearly explained what I wanted—to avoid talking about my surgeries in the lab or clinic—but I was still surprised that I didn't want to discuss it with my colleagues. There is certainly a difference between privacy and secrecy. I wasn't trying to be secretive about anything. But I also didn't want to spend my days discussing all the details with everyone I worked with. I wanted everyone who could be affected by the information to have it, but not for it to turn into a soap opera.

Facing Medical Uncertainty

There are times when doctors can be absolutely certain about a person's risk level and about the best avenue of treatment, but this is rare. Most of the time, there is considerable uncertainty about what the actual risk is for any particular person with a mutation. It depends partly on environment and your family history and, probably, on the presence of other, as-yet-undiscovered mutations that might modify the risks associated with the first mutation. There are also some newly discovered genes and mutations that are associated with a modestly higher-than-normal cancer risk, but these haven't been studied long enough for us to know just how much higher. Our catalog of these "lower-risk" genes, ones we don't understand very well, is multiplying as we learn more about human genetics.

This means that when you choose how to manage your risk, you will have to accept the fact that the data are limited. You have to do the best you can with the facts as they're currently known. For some people, this is a situation that provokes high levels of anxiety. When we see patients who are agonizing over their decision, we feel for them and also respect that they are wrestling with tough choices. I express my confidence that they will come to a choice that is best for them. The counselors and I also emphasize that making decisions is usually a process, not an event, and it happens one small step at a time.

I'm more worried when patients use the absence of data as an excuse for head-spinning denial. "My sister only had a touch of leukemia, so that's good. Now you say you can't be sure that I'll definitely get cancer, right?" they say. "Well, then I'm probably going to be fine. That's great news! Thanks for letting me know! Bye-bye!" When this happens, the genetic counselors and I are in the odd position of trying to *increase* patients' anxiety, trying to increase their ability to hear us. We want them to feel a healthy level of concern, one that motivates them to assess the facts and make a conscious, thoughtful decision. Many health professionals, including me, have frequently noticed that the lower the risk of cancer, the more anxiety a person tends to experience.

When it came time for me to make my decisions, it helped that I had a high-risk combination: a nasty mutation, a big family history of cancer, and a personal history of cancer (thankfully, it too was just a "touch" of melanoma). It was clear to me that I needed to take action. Nevertheless, I still encountered uncertainty. What were the best procedures to have? Should I have multiple procedures at the same time or separately? Where should I have them done? Should I book with the surgeon with the best technical reputation, or a surgeon known for having a human touch? Should I get reconstructive surgery?

In 2010, the British medical journal *Lancet* published an essay by Caroline Wellbery, a professor in the Department of Family Medicine at Georgetown University, about the value of medical uncertainty. Although some people see uncertainty as a problem to be resolved, Wellbery points out that this attitude isn't universal. In the arts, ambiguity is highly prized. It shows a certain respect for the facts as we know them and for those we don't yet know. It allows us to experiment with different frames, to see a situation in all its dimensions. It allows for hope. Back in physician-scientist school I'd learned that ambiguity is woven into the tapestry of medicine. The only thing that's certain is . . . uncertainty. That's what makes medicine—and life—so interesting. There's never a single right answer. There is meaning in facing uncertainty, and even in the aftermath of learning about my mutation, I felt that excitement along with the worry.

Sorting through Conflicting Information

Dealing with the uncertainty of "we don't know" is not as frustrating as dealing with conflicting recommendations from different health professionals. But conflicting recommendations happen, and you should be ready for them. For example, one of our patients came in for counseling and testing after her sister had developed breast cancer. She was found to have a BRCA2 mutation; together with her family history, we estimated that she had around a 43 percent lifetime risk for breast cancer and a 20 percent lifetime risk for ovarian cancer. She consulted a gynecological oncologist who recommended that she have her ovaries removed but not her uterus. She went for a second opinion, and the second oncologist recommended removing her uterus along with the ovaries. Which doctor, she wondered, was right?

You often hear that medicine is an art, not a science, and it's true. Sometimes there is no right or wrong. In our patient's case, the first doctor may have been thinking, "Hmmm, a possible side effect of surgery is depression. And this patient has a history of depression that is severe and long-lasting. A hysterectomy isn't necessary, so let's avoid it." The second doctor was thinking, "Let's go for all the surgeries that could prevent this patient from developing cancer. Even though the genetic risk for endometrial cancer is not thought to be that much higher than normal, let's not take that chance." Ask your doctors to lay out their reasoning, and your own choice may be easier. You can also get third and fourth and fifth opinions to see if you can draw out more information.

Choosing among Equal Options

I just talked about what happens when different doctors have different opinions, but what happens when your doctor offers you a choice? You may face a choice between two or more risk-management options that each could be appropriate. Take standard mammography. Your doctor may explain that there are choices. The American Cancer Society currently recommends that all women have annual screenings starting at age forty; the U.S. Preventive Services Task Force recommends women of normal risk have screenings starting at age fifty and every other year thereafter. A fortysomething woman with normal risk could reasonably choose either path. If you follow the American Cancer Society recommendation, you end up with a lot more trips to the doctor and could have unnecessary biopsies, but you may also derive peace of mind from undergoing more aggressive screening. If you follow the Preventive Services Task Force's guidelines, you have fewer trips to the doctor and a lower risk of false positives, but a very rare cancer might be missed. When health choices offer roughly equal advantages and disadvantages, you have an opportunity to know more about yourself. How much do you value the peace of mind? How stressful would you find the unnecessary biopsies? I've made a few of these choices myself.

Equal-options example #1: Breast reconstruction versus no reconstruction. Some women say that reconstruction has a positive emotional effect; for others, reconstruction means more surgery and more fuss. I interviewed several breast surgeons, and one mentioned—almost as an aside—that implants were more convenient than prostheses, which either stick to the chest wall or fit into a section of a special bra. In that moment, I realized that I cared about convenience. A lot. Suddenly, the hard decision became easy, and I voted for the implants. But many women choose to live with a flat chest. One of our patients was a busy CEO, and neither the longer recovery time nor waiting for a plastic surgeon appealed to her. She also didn't want to risk infection, reconstruction failure, or additional surgeries. And, she pointed out, she could always change her mind in the future.

Equal-options example #2: Surgeon X versus surgeon Y. Once I'd decided to have reconstructive surgery, I had to decide which surgeon to use. I did my due diligence. I talked with a few of each surgeon's previous patients; I asked for before-and-after photos; I had the doctors answer all the technical questions on my list and Sean's list. Both surgeons were excellent. But one surgeon talked about the procedure in a careful, conservative way; the other was more confident and his answers were less detailed. When I chose the first doctor, I had another realization: I may be a Pollyanna at heart, but I like my doctors to be cautious.

When you are faced with equal choices, you get to more clearly define who you are. I discovered that I am for convenience and medical conservatism—and in the years since the surgeries I've also realized that I am for exercise, love, peace, and people taking their own paths. I'm also sometimes for working until I burn out, taking things personally, and competing when it's not necessary. It's freeing to know that I have values that define me. Far from being a source of agony and dread, hard choices are an opportunity for us to celebrate what is so good and interesting about solving problems.

Managing External Pressures

When you're trying to decide what's best for you, pressure from other people—whether friends, family, or society in general—can be particularly troublesome. A common complaint we hear from patients is that when they start taking *any* steps toward managing the risk of inherited cancer, their families get agitated. These are the families that also don't want to think about cancer or talk about cancer or acknowledge that cancer is running through their family tree. The relatives try to guilt-trip our patients. The family members cry that they are "stirring up the pot." But that's how families stay healthy. Stirring the pot isn't a bad thing. Otherwise, the soup gets cold and congealed. Don't let the pressure get to you. Tell yourself that it's your turn to hold the spoon.

I've seen women whose husbands pressure them to reject mastectomies, for purely selfish reasons. They don't want their wives to change. My take? If someone is pushing you to make a choice that they know is bad for your health, it's time to reconsider the relationship. But some spouses and friends and siblings object to preventive surgeries because they don't understand the logic. Or they can't comprehend the statistics. Why, they wonder, would you undergo a major surgery when you don't have a cancer diagnosis? These people care about you; to them, the surgery seems drastic and unnecessary. Talk to them about the reasons for your decision. If emotions are running high, send them information via email or have your doctor send a link or attachment they can read. Give them time to think about and come to terms with your choice. Just don't let their lack of understanding sway your decision.

Tools for Resolving Decisional Conflict

For any of the reasons above, you may feel decisional conflict. Several strategies can be used to resolve the conflict and make decisions with confidence.

GET COMFORTABLE WITH IMPERFECT CHOICES AND OUTCOMES

Because you can't know the future, you're rarely going to feel that there is a single perfect choice or outcome. If you can become comfortable with this imperfection, you'll be able to make a better choice. When I had to make my risk-management decisions, I was already packing some experience in this area of imperfect choices.

By the time I was a teenager, I had made my peace with the violin, and then some. I wanted to be a concert violinist. I'd even joined my brother Tony as a performance major at Indiana University's School of Music, and for a few years I spent most of my time practicing, learning music theory and history, and taking some high-school correspondence courses. I enjoyed the life of a music student, but as time went on, it became clear that Tony (and one of our classmates, Joshua Bell) was on a trajectory to greatness, whereas my star was of a more mediocre wattage. When Tony won a bronze medal in the famous International Tchaikovsky Competition in Moscow, he returned to Indiana and played a welcome-home recital to wave after wave of standing ovations. I was happy for Tony, but I realized that I had to make a tough decision. If I stuck with the violin, I knew I would never be the musician that he was (and is). If I gave up the violin, I'd lose my life in music.

I quit music altogether. I had no idea what was on the other side of that choice; I just decided that I didn't want to be a mediocre musician. I left school, went home to Kalamazoo, and somehow snared a job as a clerk at the Kalamazoo Public Library. I mourned the loss of my violin studies, but I was starting again, and it was the first time in my life that I was comfortable with uncertainty. The act of making an imperfect choice left me exhilarated. I taught myself the "one day at a time" mantra while I figured out the next steps.

You have probably had to make some imperfect decisions in your life, too. You may even feel some satisfaction in the way you handled them. Now you may have to decide between living with risk or having preventative surgeries. You may have to choose between undergoing surgery now, when it might disrupt your life plans, or having it later, even though there's a chance you could develop cancer in the meantime. Neither option is perfect, but acknowledging that imperfection can give you the confidence to weigh your medical options and decide.

KNOW YOUR FLAWS IN PERCEPTION

Understanding your limitations can help in your decision making. Know where you tend to go wrong. How do you get fooled? For example, I'm an optimist, sometimes to an extreme. When I was considering having my uterus removed, I looked at my family tree to understand my risk. I saw Grammy's endometrial cancer—and I said to myself, "Oh, that's *nothing*! I'm sure I won't get that." My reasoning reminds me of the patient who told one of our genetic counselors that her relative had a "teaspoon of cancer." Nothing to worry about!

I keep on the sunny side. *Way* over on the sunny side. That's why I force myself to confer with people like Sean, who can size up a situation and immediately produce a list of all the things that can go wrong. He's my balancer. He's the one who would remind me to ask: What's the average recovery time for implant reconstruction compared to that for flap reconstruction (which usually takes tissue from the abdomen and uses it to reconstruct the breasts)? What's the chance that there's already a breast or ovarian cancer developing, and if there is, what's the plan?

And mind you, I was not perfectly successful in my decision making. I decided not to have my uterus removed, and I felt the negative consequences of this decision. In the years after the surgeries to remove my breasts and ovaries, I had several endometrial biopsies that showed abnormal cells, ones that threated to turn into cancer, before I finally asked the gynecologist to just take the uterus out. I should have had it removed sooner. Since Grammy (and maybe Aunt Evie) had endometrial cancer, it didn't make sense for me to play around.

MAKE ONLY THE IMPORTANT DECISIONS

Making big choices can be exhausting. Save up your decision-making power for the ones that really count. Be choosy about choosing. Let someone else decide what to make for dinner. Wear the same damn outfit to work every day if that makes things easier. Stick with your current cable-Internet-phone bundle, even if a new company wants you to compare and save costs. This way, you'll have energy to make the really big decisions and to face decisional conflict with all the strength you can muster.

CONDITION YOURSELF FOR
COMPLEX DECISIONS

In a 1995 study published in the *Journal of the American Medical Association*, Dr. Donald Redelmeier and psychologist Eldar Shafir showed a group of orthopedists a case study about an aging farmer. The farmer had right hip pain that was worsening. The investigators invited the physicians to imagine themselves as the farmer's doctor, saying, "You have tried several . . . anti-inflammatory agents [for this patient] and have stopped them because of either adverse effects or lack of efficacy. You decide to refer him . . . for hip replacement surgery."

To half the physicians, the investigators added this twist: "Before sending him away, however, you check the drug formulary and find that there is one [medication] not tried (ibuprofen). What do you do?" Most of the doctors said they'd put a hold on surgery and try the more conservative ibuprofen route first.

The other half of the group received this information: "Before sending him away, however, you check the drug formulary and find that there are two [medications] not tried (ibuprofen and piroxicam). What do you do?"

The second group faced a decision that was more complex. These doctors had to decide whether to put a hold on surgery, *and* they had to decide which of the two medications to try. What did the doctors decide? The majority of physicians in the second group chose to recommend having the hip replaced. In essence, and unconsciously, they avoided having to make a complicated decision.

Risk-management decisions have a way of getting complicated, fast. Do you want a full or a partial colectomy? Do you want to have a hysterectomy, too? At the same time or separately? Since our new hospital is almost ready to open, do you want to postpone surgery until construction is complete? Do you want to save up money in your health savings account first? While you're at it, shouldn't you get that weird mole on your neck looked at as well? There are three dermatologists within a five-mile radius of your house. Which one do you want to see?

The farmer study showed that when people are faced with complex decisions, they default to the option that requires the least thought. Don't let this happen to you, and don't cave in to pressure to decide quickly. You can always say to a doctor (or a partner or parent or friend who is pressing you for a fast decision), "I see that I have several decisions to make here. I'll need some time to think them through. Can I get back to you with questions?" Untangle the decisions. Put them into categories (a process described later in this chapter). Make each decision as separate from the others as possible.

You can also condition yourself for complexity by taking things slowly. One of our patients knew about her family history of Lynch syndrome, but when she thought about testing for the specific mutation in the family *and* getting a colonoscopy to look for colon cancer *and* deciding about preventive surgeries, her mind went blank. The possibilities and choices overwhelmed her. Eventually, though, she decided to do *just one thing*. She had a colonoscopy. The test found a large polyp, but, thank goodness, no full-blown Lynch syndrome cancer. Having taken that step, she decided to be tested for the mutation. It came back positive. Now she's reviewing her options for surgery to prevent the endometrial and ovarian cancers that are associated with the syndrome. Some people might argue that she's moved too slowly. Maybe that's true. But she *is* moving steadily, one step and one decision at a time, and that's better than not making progress at all.

MAKE YOUR OPTIONS CONCRETE

To understand the options in front of you, make them as concrete as possible. When I was deciding about reconstructive breast surgery, one of my doctors showed me a book of before and after photos. I was able to gaze at the results and see that they were likely better than what I was starting with (who among us has the perfect set?). I also asked about the specific cosmetic and physical differences between implants and flap surgeries, which use tissue from the abdomen or, less often, other donor sites such as the back or backside to reconstruct the breasts. TRAM (transverse rectus abdominis myocutaneous) flap surgeries can lead to stomach-muscle weakness, which can be a drawback for athletic women. I didn't want to lose my dream of someday playing in the LPGA!

Here are other ways to make your options concrete:

- If surgery is an option, talk to your surgeon and your surgeon's nurse. Ask for details about the surgery, healing, and aftereffects.
- Ask to speak with other patients who've had the same procedures. Ask them the same questions. How have their lives changed?
- Learn more about what could happen if you don't have surgery. What is your risk if you choose to have screenings

instead, or follow other measures? What is the likelihood that a cancer could be caught early through screenings and treated successfully? What would that treatment look like?

- Visualize yourself living *without* the surgery or procedure in question. How do you feel? How is your life different? If you have frequent screenings in place of surgery, do you have "scanxiety"—lots of dread and fear before you get the test results? How do you react if the scan finds something and you need a biopsy? Would you regret not having surgery?
- Imagine all the positive things that can happen if you live longer. Does this vision of your future affect your decision?

PUT YOUR OPTIONS INTO CATEGORIES

To make your decisions clear, sort each one into its own category. That way, you make just one decision at a time instead of feeling as if you're trapped in an endless algorithm. I found that for each surgery I was considering, there were several categories of questions:

Whether **to have the surgery.** I had a strong emotional response to this question. When it came to a mastectomy and an oophorectomy, I knew that I wanted to avoid ending up in Bea's situation, with an aggressive breast cancer at a young age. Another person may not have felt so strongly and may have decided on increased surveillance (mammography and MRI) or a course of tamoxifen. But as I mentioned above, when I thought about uterine removal, I chose to pass. As I also mentioned, I eventually reversed that decision. Your age may factor into this decision as well. Younger individuals who are mutation positive may decide on intensive surveillance at first while they find their life partners and decide whether or not to have biological children. These decisions may be quite complicated for very young women. For example, consider a patient who finds out she has a BRCA1 mutation at age twenty.

She finds herself staying in imperfect relationships as she subconsciously strives to be married with children as soon as possible. She's conflicted by her desire for children and her need to have her ovaries removed before age thirty-five. She has nagging questions. Would it be harder to date with scars? When do you tell your boyfriend about your mutation? Will he stay with you when he finds out?

Where **to have the surgery.** I was choosing between home in Ann Arbor and Boston, where I'd done my internship and residency. I chose Boston, mostly for the privacy and because close friends lived there. When choosing between hospitals in Boston, no neurons were needed—I simply went where my chosen group of surgeons practiced their art: Brigham and Women's Hospital.

When **to have the surgery.** Should I delay until a more convenient time or have it right away? For me, this was easy: I wanted surgery as soon as possible. I didn't want to get a cancer while waiting. Other people might decide to take their time and undergo surveillance for a few years while they get used to knowing that they carry a cancer mutation.

Who **should do the surgery.** I interviewed several doctors over the phone and then chose among them based on their availability and their skills. Others might have chosen the surgeon based just on their skills and not cared about waiting for them to become available.

How **to have the surgery.** Should I have one that combined mastectomies and oophorectomies, or do them in two stages? I chose to do them in two stages to avoid prolonged anesthesia. Others may have preferred it in one stage to get it all over with—like yanking off a Band-Aid as opposed to peeling it off slowly.

You'll have your own categories, of course. Categories need to speak to your own way of thinking, not that of your doctor or your partner.

Even when a medical decision is really important, it can be OK to punt—to let someone you trust make the decision. Yes, this means that the decision is no longer yours. Yes, the decision could turn out to be the wrong one for you. But if you're exhausted and need to hand over a few choices, you shouldn't feel guilty. When my old mentor from Harvard sent Sean and me an email about freezing eggs prior to surgery, I decided to pass this decision on to Sean. I was uncertain and tired, but for Sean the decision was a no-brainer. We had a full life as it was. His willingness to make a choice for us, and to take the responsibility for that choice, comforted me. I didn't have to make all the hard decisions on my own.

Not that I didn't have regrets. Later, I found myself obsessed with not being able to have biological children. This wasn't entirely logical. I had a great but demanding job and a great but still-young family. The possibility of actually being able to handle more children was one of my fantasies. Still, I spent a lot of time trying to meditate myself out of a state of sadness, and not always succeeding. I finally got a boot out of my funk when our girls became teenagers. They were more independent, and I started to enjoy having more time for work. My desire for more children faded.

If I could go back in time, would I have done things differently and frozen my eggs? Maybe, but nobody is perfect. Hard choices are hard because there is no right answer. Earlier in this chapter, I said that hard choices give you the opportunity to learn about yourself, to define yourself. Among other things, I learned that it's possible for me to run out of juice—to find myself too spent to make one more decision. When this happened, I was grateful to have Sean step in and make that decision for me. I still am.

Chapter Seven

Targeted Treatments for Cancer:
Realities, Myths, Possibilities

IN THE LATE 1800s, two Appalachian families were locked in a bitter, murderous feud. There were knife fights, gunfights, and outright executions. The names of these families—Hatfield and McCoy—are so infamous that they have become a metaphor for old-time violence. But let's think about one of these families in terms of something that's relatively new: targeted treatments for cancer.

From 1964 to 1994, researchers at the University of Virginia's general research center in Charlottesville studied and cared for four generations of the McCoy family. They found something unusual, even stunning. More than seventeen members of the family had pheochromocytomas (the same rare adrenal gland tumors that both Grumpy and Ms. Adora had). Even more remarkable, each McCoy who had one of these tumors also had a mutation in the VHL gene, giving them a diagnosis of Von Hippel–Lindau syndrome. People with this inherited cancer syndrome are more likely to get pheochromocytomas as well as kidney cancers and vascular tumors of the eye and nervous system.

The researchers published the family's genetic information in 1998, calling them the "McC kindred" to preserve their privacy. In 2007, McCoy family members took their story public, speaking to the press so that distant relatives might learn about their risk for Von Hippel–Lindau syndrome and get the screenings that could save their lives. When the story broke, historians were aflutter. Why? Because pheochromocytomas can lead to behavioral changes, including adrenaline-fueled aggressiveness—a trait that was a hallmark of the feuding family. When pheochromocytomas are surgically removed, personalities return to normal. (The surgery also prevents the tumor from causing a stroke or even death.) What if the nineteenth-century feuding McCoys could have been screened for VHL mutations and treated? Would they have been less quick to draw their weapons? Would they have made peace with the Hatfields? It's possible. It's fun to speculate.

Today, people with a known VHL mutation have a brand-new treatment option. If they develop advanced kidney cancer, they can take drugs that are tailored specifically to their cancer's molecular abnormalities, including drugs with the difficult-to-pronounce names of sunitinib (trade name Sutent) or sorafenib (Nexavar). The drugs on their own don't cure the cancers, but sometimes they can downgrade them into something resembling a chronic, manageable disorder.

Sunitinib and sorafenib are examples of what are known as molecularly targeted therapies for cancer: They are therapies that take aim at individual molecules that cancers need to survive, grow, and spread. It's not as if there is a single predictable set of molecules that appears in all cancers. Doctors often explain cancer by saying, "It's not just one disease. It's more than a hundred diseases." I do the same. But now it seems possible that the reason cancer is so hard to treat is that everyone's cancer is a little bit different. As the science reporter George Johnson says in his book *The Cancer Chronicles,* cancer could be hundreds of thousands of diseases, or millions. In the future, after we are better able to interpret genetic data, it may become useful to know everything about each cancer's genetics, including genetic inheritance and family history, as well as the genetic changes that occur in the tumor itself.

Up until this point in the book, I've talked about the ways genetic knowledge can reduce your cancer risk. Here, I'll show you how genetic knowledge may influence your treatment if you do get cancer. I'll explain how mutations in the germline genome (which are the genes that you have inherited from your parents) and the tumor genome (the genes you have inherited from your parents *plus* additional "somatic" mutations that occur only in the cancer cells) can be used to inform treatment plans. I will tell you in general terms what we know about molecular targeting of tumors and the tumor-associated immune system. I won't try to discuss every new oncology drug or all the caveats that must be considered when using them.

The germline mutations that are inherited from your parents are identified by sequencing the DNA in your normal cells—commonly cells from your saliva or blood. This will identify mutations that predispose to cancer, such as those in the VHL and BRCA genes. Sometimes identification of these mutations influences cancer treatment and sometimes it does not. Most commonly, germline DNA is sequenced not to guide cancer treatment strategies but to assess whether you have a genetic predisposition to cancer. That is, as we've discussed, to devise prevention strategies.

In contrast, somatic mutations that occur in cancer cells can be identified only by sequencing the DNA in cancer cells after a tumor has been detected. This is done to identify the mutations that are driving the growth of the cancer. When cancer cells are sequenced, the hope is that mutations will be found against which targeted therapies are available. That allows physicians to customize therapies to go after some of the specific molecules that are driving cancer growth in specific patients. Unfortunately, our armamentarium of targeted therapies remains limited—we don't yet have drugs that target many of the mutant genes that drive cancer growth. Consequently, while cancers are increasingly being sequenced in an effort to predict their clinical behaviors (cancers with different combinations of mutations are known to behave differently and to respond differently to therapies of all kinds), patients still have to get "lucky" by having a mutation against which a targeted therapy is available.

The McCoy family is our prototype for why genetic knowledge matters for patients with a genetic cancer predisposition—and also for patients without one. Having an inherited mutation, such as the McCoy's VHL mutation, in the germline genome doesn't mean those patients get a kidney cancer that is different from the kidney cancers of patients that do not have an inherited mutation. The predisposition simply means that a patient has a head start and can come down with the same cancers earlier and more often. Germline genome mutations can certainly inform the treatment in some kinds of cancers. However, more often than not, it's additional mutations in the tumor genome and the subsequent molecular alterations in the tumor cells that guide targeted treatment strategies. I'll take a look at the research that is pursuing targeted and so-called personalized treatments, including hormonal therapies and therapies known as kinase inhibitors and PARP inhibitors, and even touch on the recent promise of immune therapies. Most important, I'll help you separate the hope from the hype.

What Are Targeted Therapies?

The goal of targeted therapies is to eradicate cancer cells with limited side effects. When I was an oncology fellow, one of my clinical teachers told us to think of cancers as dandelions that take root in your yard and then spread. (He said the same thing to his patients, who may not have found the analogy as endearing as we did.) Traditional cancer therapies try to cut out or dig up the dandelions (surgery), burn the dandelions (radiation), or poison the dandelions (chemotherapy). Cut, burn, poison—it sounds like a horror movie. And as with the action in a horror movie, these therapies are harsh. Just as cutting, burning, or poisoning your dandelions will unavoidably harm some of the healthy grass in your yard, undergoing surgery, radiation, or chemotherapy will also harm the cells around the cancer. And although surgery, radiation, and chemotherapy can be successful, in many cancers they're not successful often enough. Targeted therapies are an attempt to address these shortcomings. By administering a drug that inhibits a specific protein that cancer cells need more than normal cells do, molecularly targeted therapies can kill the cancer cells without killing normal cells. In theory, targeted therapies could kill just the dandelions—or prevent them from reproducing—and leave the rest of the yard green and thriving.

Consider chemotherapy, for example. Chemotherapy works largely because it hits cells that are rapidly dividing. There are a few problems, though. Not all rapidly dividing cells are cancer cells. Some are normal cells in highly regenerative tissues (in which cells are regularly replaced by new cells), such as those found in the lining of your intestines, the blood-forming system, and hair follicles. That's why people typically lose their hair during chemotherapy and their blood cell counts have to be monitored carefully. And not all cancer cells divide rapidly. Some divide more slowly, and these cells can survive chemotherapy. In contrast, targeted treatments inhibit specific proteins within cells. Often, these are mutant forms of proteins that are present only in the cancer cells. So, molecularly targeted therapies are designed to do a better job of killing cancer cells with fewer side effects on normal cells.

When you hear people talk about targeted therapies, you will often hear the phrase "personalized medicine" or "precision medicine." Doctors have always been trained to personalize cancer therapies for their patients. For example, they may time a treatment so that the patient can energetically attend a special event, like a wedding. When a patient suffers from a severe side effect of treatment, good doctors consider a different treatment or ways to reduce the side effect.

However, "personalized medicine" can also refer to a new wave of research into targeted therapies that could address the specific molecular profile in a patient's cancer rather than targeting the tumor with only a surgical knife or a radiation therapy's ray. This specific molecular profile is like a lock, and a personalized or targeted therapy acts as its specially made key. This is an Achilles' heel for the cancer cells because, in principle, therapies that attack mutant proteins that arise from the mutations present only in the cancer cells (the somatic mutations that are identified by tumor sequencing) can kill the cancer cells without killing normal cells. In practice, it's more complicated. Even targeted therapies can have some toxicity to normal tissues, partly by having "off-target" effects in which they bind and inhibit things they're not supposed to bind.

These "locks" and "keys" have been found in several cancers. Chronic myeloid leukemia (CML) is one of the most famous examples. This type of leukemia occurs mainly in patients without inherited cancer syndromes, with the possible exception of patients with Li-Fraumeni syndrome (TP53 mutations). The poster patient for chronic myeloid leukemia is Kareem Abdul-Jabbar, who does not have an inherited predisposition to cancer but has had this leukemia since 2008. This disease develops only when a mutated kinase called BCR-ABL is present in the tumor cells. A kinase is an enzyme that sends signals inside cells. BCR-ABL signals bone marrow cells to survive and proliferate when they shouldn't. Normally, BCR and ABL are different proteins encoded by different genes, but a mutation in the cancer cell's genome can produce a cell with a hybrid BCR-ABL gene, which will manufacture the problematic protein with extra kinase activity. Since this mutant protein is not present in normal cells, and yet is required by the cancer cells, a drug that specifically inhibits BCR-ABL would, in principle, be toxic only to the cancer cells.

Enter the drug imatinib (Gleevec), which binds to BCR-ABL and inhibits the kinase activity. Since most of the cancer cells can't survive without BCR-ABL signaling, imatinib kills the vast majority of leukemia cells with few side effects on normal cells. Abdul-Jabbar has been on imatinib since his diagnosis in 2008 and his disease remains, as he tweeted in 2011, "at a minimum." And in August 2014, he told *Parade* that he's still healthy: "I take my medication and tell everybody something else is going to have to kill me." This has been a boon not only for Abdul-Jabbar and his family and friends but also for all of us. He uses his prominence and experience to lobby for cancer research.

Although the therapy restores the health of patients, it does not cure the leukemia, because some leukemia cells survive. That means that despite regaining their health, patients like Abdul-Jabbar still have leukemia cells lurking inside, waiting to take over as soon as imatinib is stopped. Consequently, patients must stay on imatinib for the long term to suppress the development of leukemia in much the same way as patients with human immunodeficiency virus (HIV) must chronically stay on antiviral medications to suppress HIV replication. There are also instances in which imatinib works for a while, but then BCR-ABL acquires other somatic mutations in cancer cells so that it no longer binds the drug; fortunately, there are additional drugs to use when this happens. These drugs have transformed CML from a disease that required a bone marrow transplant to avoid a certain death into a chronic disease, in some ways similar to how diabetes was transformed into a chronic disease by insulin. Although many (not all) patients can be alive and healthy with CML and diabetes for many years, there remains much room for improvement; medical scientists continue to seek a cure for both. As you'll see, there are reasons to be hopeful about the future of targeted therapies, but the road won't be easy or short.

Targeted cancer treatments can be lumped into three major categories. The first category is that of hormone therapies such as tamoxifen for breast cancer or anti-androgens for prostate cancer. The second is small-molecule inhibitors; they can slide into cancer cells, bind to specific target proteins inside the cells, and inactivate them. Usually, these drugs inhibit the enzymatic activity (e.g., kinase or DNA repair activity) of a protein that's necessary for cancer cell survival. You can spot these drugs easily: Their generic names commonly end in "-ib," for the second syllable of "inhibitor." Imatinib, the drug that is keeping Kareem Abdul-Jabbar's leukemia at bay, is a case in point. Beyond hormone therapies and the small-molecule enzyme inhibitors, the third major class of targeted agents is therapeutic monoclonal antibodies, or "-mabs" for short. These antibodies target specific proteins on the surfaces of cancer or immune cells.

Hormonal Therapies

Tamoxifen, the first targeted cancer treatment, is a terrific example of how molecularly targeted treatments pinpoint a cancer's "bull's-eye." But it also shows why cancer cures are so elusive. You can give a patient a targeted treatment, but sometimes the target will move.

In the 1970s and '80s, breast cancer research took advantage of a new piece of knowledge: Not all breast cancers, it turned out, are the same. Some breast tumors have estrogen receptors (ERs)—a clue that the cancers are being fueled by estrogen. When estrogen binds to ERs inside the cancer cells, the receptors are turned on; they turn on genes that tell the cells to survive and proliferate.

Tamoxifen blocks that action by binding to ERs and blocking the receptors from binding estrogen. Tamoxifen dethrones estrogen by taking estrogen's seat at the estrogen receptor table. Sorry, estrogen, you can't sit here! In breast cancer cells this prevents ER signaling, depriving the cells of survival and proliferation signals. From many years of clinical experience, we know now that when patients with ER-positive cancers take tamoxifen after they've had surgery to remove the primary tumor, it reduces the chance of cancer recurrence by 50 percent. By 1993, when Grammy was diagnosed with breast cancer, tamoxifen was the standard of care for women with ER-positive breast cancers.

Grammy took tamoxifen every day for five years. Only *half* the breast cancer patients who start on tamoxifen—recall, it's a drug that has been proven to cut the rate of cancer recurrence by 50 percent—keep up their regimens. One of the reasons is that tamoxifen has side effects that some patients find difficult. Tamoxifen is much less harsh than chemotherapy, but it's no walk in the park, either. It can lead to hot flashes, mood swings, and, very rarely, endometrial cancer and blood clots. Yet Grammy's breast cancer was cured by surgery, radiation, and tamoxifen.

By taking tamoxifen, Grammy has also likely prevented new breast cancers from developing. Tamoxifen was the drug our young BRCA1 mutant patient (described in chapter 6) took to reduce her risk while she decided whether and when to have prophylactic surgeries. The idea is that if a woman is at high risk for breast cancer because of a family history or having a known cancer gene mutation, tamoxifen can reduce the risk of future cancers. This insight was born from data. When treating patients for their breast tumors with tamoxifen, oncologists observed that the women who, like Grammy, completed a five-year course of tamoxifen had fewer breast cancers than expected in the opposite breast. Studies have confirmed that tamoxifen reduces risk in high-risk patients. It's possible that tamoxifen keeps microscopic pre-cancers from developing into cancer by impairing their survival and proliferation.

Hormonal therapies are also used against other cancers, prostate cancer in particular. But a patient can develop resistance to hormonal therapy's effects. Some breast cancers respond at first to tamoxifen, but then the tumor adapts to the drug and stops responding—either the tumor learns how to proliferate in the absence of ER signaling or the ER no longer binds to tamoxifen. In fact there is considerable heterogeneity within tumors, with different combinations of mutations in different cells. This leads to natural selection within tumors, as cells with deleterious (to the cancer cell) mutations die off and cells with advantageous mutations outcompete other cells. This means that when cancer cells are subject to a strong selective pressure, like drug treatment, the cells that are sensitive to the drug die, and the cells with mutations that confer drug resistance survive to regrow the tumors. As a consequence of this constant selection for increasingly "fit" cancer cells, cancers become increasingly aggressive and less responsive to therapy over time.

Research into hormonal therapies continues, and so does research into other targeted drugs that may be able to step in when a tumor develops resistance to drugs like tamoxifen. Fulvestrant (Faslodex) binds to the ER and destroys it. Another class of drugs called aromatase inhibitors—including the medications anastrozole (Arimidex), letrozole (Femara), and exemestane (Aromasin)—decrease the amount of estrogen in the body by inhibiting its production. This deprives breast cancer cells of estrogen in a way that is similar to what happens when ovaries are surgically removed in oophorectomies.

Fulvestrant and aromatase inhibitors are already approved by the Food and Drug Administration (FDA) and available to patients. Researchers are also testing new drugs that inhibit enzymes or secondary targets that are involved in hormone-therapy resistance.

A top secondary target is a molecule called phosphatidylinositol 3-kinase (PI3-kinase), which can send signals in cancer cells that replace the need for estrogen receptor signals. By blocking PI3-kinase, we hope to outsmart the cancer. We'll need more drugs that can block cancer's ability to reinvent itself. In the future, we have to go beyond understanding a person's current cancer; we have to figure out ways to be one step ahead and predict cancer's next moves.

Kinase Inhibitors

The drug that Abdul-Jabbar takes for his leukemia, imatinib, is a small-molecule kinase inhibitor. Kinases send signals inside cells by chemically modifying other proteins, which changes their structure and function. When Grumpy was fighting his final bout with lung cancer, he tried a kinase inhibitor called gefitinib (Iressa). All that happened was he got a bad case of acne—at age eighty-three. It gave him something to joke about, but we were all disappointed that the drug didn't work.

At the same time, I was caring for a breast cancer patient whose husband, Larry, developed the same kind of lung cancer as Grumpy's. Larry was so sick that he was unable to get out of bed. Then he took gefitinib and felt so much better that he was able to spend hours in the Michigan woods, hunting deer with his son. He wasn't cured, but he enjoyed a year of high-quality remission. Why didn't Grumpy get the same results from the same drug? We chalked it up to bad luck. Back then, we didn't know that Grumpy and Larry had the same kind of cancer caused by different mutations. While Larry's mutation conferred sensitivity to gefitinib, unfortunately Grumpy's did not.

Gefitinib was on the market for a while before we learned why some lung cancer patients like Larry had such extraordinary remissions and others didn't. It works on tumors that make a mutated form of a kinase called EGFR (also known as HER1). When Larry took gefitinib, his mutated kinase was inhibited, and his tumor melted away. Not completely, but significantly. Grumpy's tumor didn't have the EGFR mutation; gefitinib couldn't fix what wasn't broken.

Targeted drugs are often developed by finding targets in cancer cells and *then* creating drugs against them. But this usually doesn't fully explain why some cancers respond and some do not. Over the years, we were able to more precisely define the target that gefitinib was acting on, and only then could we match the treatment to the person. Successful research rarely moves in a straight line. You have to allow room for creative stumbling, serendipity, and old-fashioned trial and error.

Kinase inhibitor research goes beyond targeted treatments for lung and breast cancers. The drug imatinib, the one that's shown great success against chronic myeloid leukemia, is a product of that research. Scientists are also looking closely at a particularly interesting target, vascular endothelial growth factor (VEGF) receptors. Sunitinib and sorafinib, the "-ib" drugs used against kidney cancer in those with Von Hippel-Lindau syndrome, like the McCoys', or those without a known inherited cancer syndrome, work by inhibiting the VEGF receptor in their tumor cells. And a multi-kinase inhibitor named vandetanib helps patients who develop medullary thyroid cancer. Vandetanib targets the VEGF receptor and other kinases that are hyperactive in hereditary medullary thyroid cancers driven by RET mutations.

As an example, a recent young patient of ours was diagnosed with medullary thyroid cancer and subsequently found to have an inherited RET mutation similar to Ms. Adora's mutation. Although she and several of her family members with the RET mutation have now had their thyroids removed to prevent additional cancers, it's possible that remnants of her tumor are still in her body and she will need further treatment. Vandetanib will be an option for her. If her cancer returns, this new therapy has a good chance of making her future longer and healthier.

PARP Inhibitors

Every day, every cell in your body takes a hit to its DNA, as little breaks occur along its strands. These breaks cause the mutations that can predispose to cancer. In the early 1990s, scientists discovered that an enzyme called poly ADP ribose polymerase (thankfully abbreviated as PARP) helps repair those breaks, like an electrician called out to repair damaged wires after a storm. Radiation therapy is like one of those storms. Radiation therapy fragments cellular DNA so effectively that cancer cells die. Unfortunately, high levels of radiation can also kill the patient by fragmenting the DNA of cells in certain normal tissues like blood-forming cells and cells that line the inside of your intestine, so the rays can't be deployed at full strength. As a result, many but not all cancer cells are killed. When PARP's repairing activity was discovered, scientists wondered whether inhibiting PARP activity would increase the number of irradiated cancer cells that are killed by preventing them from repairing the DNA damage.

You may be wondering whether PARP inhibitors or radiation can also cause new cancers by preventing normal cells from repairing their DNA. This is a concern, but normal cells have backup repair systems that some cancer cells lack, and the doses are carefully selected to reduce the risks of therapy-induced cancers. Moreover, PARP inhibitors can work a kind of pharmaceutical jujitsu—they can preferentially kill cancer cells by exploiting some of the very mutations that cause them.

Tumors with BRCA mutations, for example, are unable to fix certain kinds of complex breaks in both DNA strands. Each position in your chromosomes has two complementary strands of DNA bound to each other. When mutations affect only a single strand, they are easy to repair because the correct information can be copied from the intact complementary strand. Other mutations affect both strands. These so-called double-strand breaks are more complex to repair because the information on both strands has been corrupted. Cancer cells usually don't have to fix many double-strand breaks, because PARP repairs single-strand breaks before they progress to double-strand breaks. By inhibiting PARP, the tumor loses its first line of defense. And a tumor with a BRCA mutation doesn't have a second line of defense. Thus, when treated with a PARP inhibitor, a tumor cell is defenseless to repair itself after irradiation. The cell dies a death of destruction and, let's hope, some well-deserved despair. (Tumors with mutations in other DNA repair genes such as PALB2 and RAD51C may be vulnerable to PARP inhibitors for a similar reason.)

Although several small-molecule PARP inhibitor cancer drugs are being developed and tested, they're on a bumpy road to the clinic. A case in point: Scientists were excited about a supposed PARP inhibitor named iniparib, which showed signs in early testing of being a superstar. In fact, an inspiring ovarian cancer patient named Dr. Carol Basbaum is the mother of all PARP inhibitors. Basbaum, who had a BRCA1 mutation, was an accomplished scientist who worked at the University of California, San Francisco, as the "queen of mucous." For years she and her laboratory experimentally dissected how our lungs keep us safe. After her ovarian cancer diagnosis, her morning and night jobs were to push iniparib into the clinic. Although Basbaum died from her ovarian cancer before PARP inhibitors were tested in people, she ignited the first phases of the PARP-inhibitor field.

After getting deep into the clinical testing process, the company testing iniparib in patients, Sanofi announced that, based on its late-stage trial results, it was going to discontinue work on the drug. This led many researchers to stop working on PARP inhibitors altogether. If the most promising new drug didn't work, they asked themselves, why bother investigating any of the others? The field paused. Then, in a twist, scientists who were working independently of Sanofi reported that in cultured cells, iniparib did not appear to be a standard PARP inhibitor after all. It now seems possible that iniparib could still be a successful drug, as some patients have benefited on the trials. It just might not be a standard PARP inhibitor, and it might not work on the cancers that Sanofi initially tested it on. Iniparib is now, like gefitinib was in 2003, a potential solution looking for a problem.

Basbaum fought and researched ovarian cancer for more than five years before her death. She was treated with the usual surgery and chemotherapy; successive chemotherapies worked and then stopped. How she was able to keep the cancer in check while tolerating chemotherapies and producing great research for so long is a mystery. Did her love for science keep her immune system revved up? We'll never know. What we do know is that a promising "targeted" drug for ovarian cancer wasn't available to her—but certainly not for the lack of trying.

This promising new drug was not available to her because it was only in 2014, almost ten years after Basbaum's death, that PARP inhibitor research took an important step into the clinic. Olaparib (Lynparza), another PARP inhibitor, was approved by the FDA for use in patients who have BRCA mutations and advanced ovarian cancer. It's the first PARP inhibitor approved for clinical use, and the approval is conditional. If the next phase (phase III; I'll define the phases later in the chapter) of testing doesn't show a good outcome, we're back to square one—and back to having no PARP inhibitors on the market. This would not be an uncommon result. When phase II trials are promising but later-stage, controlled phase

III trials fail to show safety or efficacy, there is deep disappointment. It's a harsh reality check.

Olaparib has also been proposed as a possible cancer-prevention pill, similar to tamoxifen, for use in patients at high risk for cancer, such as those with BRCA mutations. Researchers have found that PARP inhibition can delay the development of breast cancers in mice with BRCA1 mutations. It's important to note that the formation was delayed, not prevented. Furthermore, the potential for damage to normal tissues by long-term PARP inhibition still needs to be studied. More realistic models coupled with trials in humans still need to happen. These ideas for cancer prevention with PARP inhibitors will be refined, tested, and retested over time. Later in this chapter, I'll explain why it's so important to let the process of testing—agonizingly slow as it is—unfold.

Therapeutic Antibodies

In addition to hormonal therapies and the small-molecule inhibitors like imatinib, gefitinib, and olaparib, the third class of agents, the therapeutic monoclonal antibodies ("-mabs"), target proteins on the surfaces of cancer cells. One of the first kinase inhibitors, trastuzumab (Herceptin), falls into this category. Trastuzumab works against HER2, a kinase that is expressed at high levels on the surface of some breast cancer cells. About 20 percent of breast cancer cases are HER2 positive, meaning that the tumor cells have duplicated the HER2 gene to accumulate many copies (the jargon is "amplified"), leading to high levels of the protein.

Trastuzumab is used in combination with chemotherapy, and its entry into the clinic has significantly improved the prognosis for HER2 positive breast cancers. Without trastuzumab, 62 percent of patients experience ten years of disease-free survival; when trastuzumab is added, the survival goes up to 74 percent. Trastuzumab can also be used in metastatic breast cancer in patients who test positive for HER2, though it doesn't offer a cure for people who are in this late stage of the disease. It can, however, extend life and reduce symptoms. We need more drugs that either work better to inhibit HER2 or to find a way to get around HER2 resistance. Research teams are at work on these challenges. Therapeutic antibodies can be used to target any molecule on any cell's surface and should not be confused with immune therapies.

Immune Therapies

The body's immune system is best known for its ability to kill germs and fight infections. But it also kills cancer cells. Immune therapies, or immunotherapies, aim to activate the body's immune system to destroy cancer cells more effectively. However, some cancers acquire genetic changes that make them invisible to immune cells or have signals on their surfaces that say, in effect, "Dear immune cells, please don't destroy me." The goal of immunotherapies is to overcome the ways that cancer cells try to fool the immune system into thinking that they are not a threat.

Immunotherapies have been tested sporadically since the late 1800s, when the surgeon William Coley injected bacteria ("Coley toxins") into tumors, hoping to stimulate an inflammatory response that would kill the tumor cells. Looking back, it's hard to evaluate Coley's findings. He reported anecdotes of patients whose tumors responded to the treatment, but when these Coley toxins were tested in small clinical trials and did not show beneficial activity, they became a historical footnote. Although Coley toxins are thought of as the precursor to contemporary immunotherapy, we now have a deeper knowledge of the immune system. Now there are designer immune therapies in development that target single molecules. These therapies either release the brakes on the immune system or hit its accelerator.

Let's look at the accelerators first. These drugs are, by coincidence, known as chimeric antigen receptor (or . . . wait for it . . . CARs) containing T cells. The antigen receptors on T cells are the proteins on the surface of the cells that recognize the foreign molecules that the T cell is programmed to attack. When the receptor binds to the molecule, or antigen (a fancy word for molecular structures recognized by the immune system), the T cell is activated and it kills whatever cell is carrying the antigen. Similar to when an interloper (the cancer cell) enters a secured compound, alarms sound, and the trespasser is, at a minimum, restrained by security (the immune cells). You have many different T cells in your body that specialize in fighting different kinds of harmful cells. For example, some T cells kill virally infected cells, and others kill bacterially infected cells. When you get an infection, the T cells that carry receptors designed to respond to that particular pathogen multiply in an attempt to wipe out the pathogens. Vaccines are designed to activate and expand the T cells specific for certain pathogens, like the flu virus, in advance of the infection so that your immune system is ready if you get exposed.

The immune system operates by self/non-self-recognition, attacking antigens it perceives not to be from your body. Normally, T cells are activated by foreign antigens—this allows them to attack pathogen-infected cells without attacking your normal cells. Sometimes the mutant genes in cancer cells produce mutant proteins (called neo-antigens) that appear foreign to the immune system. It's thought that surveillance for abnormal cells by the immune system is part of what protects us from the development of cancer— your immune system nips it in the bud before the cancer cell has a chance to multiply. But once a cancer evades the immune system long enough to grow a tumor, therapies are required to hyperactivate the immune system to give it a chance to defeat the cancer.

The CAR therapy begins when researchers collect T cells from the patient's blood. Then they alter the T cells by adding a gene for a chimeric antigen receptor (the CAR) that targets the specific neo-antigens on the patient's cancer cells. The modified T cells are then given back to the patient, whose immune system is now better armed to attack the cancer. For years scientists studied this approach to enhance immune activity against cancer cells with underwhelming results. However, recent breakthroughs have increased attention and interest in this area.

Clinical trials with CAR T cells have recently achieved shockingly impressive results. For example, a study published in the *New England Journal of Medicine* showed that in acute lymphoblastic leukemia, twenty-seven of thirty patients had a complete remission after treatment with CAR T cells. This is, as Uncle Jack might say, a "holy shit" kind of result. As you can imagine, companies are lined up to develop CAR therapies and investment is flooding into this area to optimize safety and efficacy, and, hopefully, to extend the results to additional cancers.

Other targeted immune therapies are designed to release the brakes on the immune system. These molecular brakes are known as checkpoint proteins, or co-receptors (because they bind to target cells along with the T cell receptor to inhibit T cell overactivity); they prevent T cells from getting so aggressive that they kill normal cells. When the immune system attacks normal tissues, it's called autoimmunity. This is what goes wrong in diseases like lupus. But in cancer treatment, blocking checkpoint proteins increases the ability of T cells to destroy tumor cells. Of course, one potential side effect is increased damage to normal tissues due to autoimmunity. If you have a life-threatening cancer, that's a risk most people are willing to take. Some people can't tolerate these therapies because of the damage they do to normal tissues, but many other patients experience remarkable long-term responses in which their tumors melt away without unacceptable inflammation in normal tissues.

The drugs ipilimumab (Yervoy), which targets a T cell coreceptor known as CTLA-4, and nivolumab (Opdivo), which targets another T cell co-receptor known as PD-1, are immunotherapies that are also therapeutic antibodies; they fit into the third category of targeted cancer drugs. They have been approved by the FDA for patients with advanced melanoma and are also in the late stages of testing for kidney and lung cancers. Several additional targeted immune therapies in the earlier stages of development also target PD-1 or molecules related to it. Although these immune-targeted T cell checkpoint therapies can lead to inflammation of the colon (colitis), kidney (nephritis), lung (pneumonitis), and liver (hepatitis), as well as endocrine tissues, the effects on cancers have been so impressive in a variety of clinical trials that the cancer research community is very excited about them. Nonetheless, much work remains to be done to optimize the use of these therapies, to maximize safety and efficacy, and to figure out which patients are most likely to benefit.

Combined Therapies

An interesting area of research is the use of targeted drugs in combination—for example, a kinase inhibitor plus a PARP inhibitor or a targeted immunotherapy. Combination therapy can get complicated. In a patient with kidney cancer, we may want to target an overactive kinase with sunitinib as well as unleash the patient's T cells with ipilimumab. We could theoretically give patients a combination of immunotherapies that work toward the same goal in different ways. Early experiments have tested combinations of immune checkpoint inhibitors (ipilimumab and nivolumab) in very-late-stage melanoma patients. Historically, most melanoma patients at this stage do not survive more than six months. Two years after taking the immune-therapy combination, 80 percent of the patients were still alive. As follow-up, a more advanced randomized, double-blind study in 2015 compared the same two-drug combination to ipilimumab alone and found that ipilimumab and nivolumab are indeed synergistic. Additional advanced trials are just beginning. Many other combination therapies are also in development.

Targeted immunotherapies are good candidates to work hand in hand with standard therapies like radiation and chemotherapy as well as kinase or PARP inhibitors. All these treatments can kill cancer cells, leaving a smaller tumor that's more exposed to the immune system—and immunotherapies. It's like going into battle: the fewer enemy soldiers, the more likely you'll prevail. Of course, not all targeted therapies work in synergy. Some combinations might even result in *worse* effects for the patient or increased side effects. Each combination will need to be put through clinical trials. As you'll see, clinical trials are our safeguard against giving patients drugs that may look promising but turn out to be ineffective or have unacceptable side effects. Ultimately, the goal is to have new drugs, either individually or in combination, that can be used after surgery to reduce the risk of cancer's recurrence—and that support the physician's oath to "do no harm."

How to Sift Hope from Hype

You may hear people talk about targeted therapies as if they are a brand-new way of treating cancer, but in fact they're not. Targeted therapies have been around since researchers first realized that tamoxifen could kill ER-positive breast cancer cells. They're also not bulletproof. Ideally, the side effects of targeted therapies aren't as bad as poisonous chemotherapies—but side effects do limit their use. And cancers are particularly good at adapting to develop resistance to targeted therapies. Still, the latest research into targeted treatments is promising. It's promising because as we understand the genetics of tumors, the number of ideas for drug targets is increasing rapidly, too. These increased numbers of ideas will hopefully correlate with increased real targets (like ER, BCR-ABL, and PARPs). Bottom line: It makes sense to hope that new targeted treatments may be less toxic than traditional treatments while achieving similar anticancer effects.

However, we have to look at targeted treatments with our eyes wide open. There are lots of ideas out there, but many drugs still need to go through clinical trials before we will know whether they are effective. I sometimes hear patients express frustration with the process of clinical trials. To them, it seems as if potentially valuable drugs are being kept from the public while being forced through a nitpicky process of being tested and retested. I understand wanting to have access to drugs that we think might work. But I also know, as a researcher and as an advocate for my sister, Bea, and my patients, that this process of clinical testing is absolutely necessary.

Medicine has a long history of new therapies that were widely expected to work but turned out not to work when carefully tested. Sometimes, people are so convinced therapies will work that physicians start using them "off-label" (for an indication other than what was approved by the FDA) before the clinical trials are done. Arthroscopic knee surgery is a recent example. Doctors were performing hundreds of thousands of these surgeries per year at a cost of more than five thousand dollars each. It seemed to relieve pain in about half the arthritis patients who had it done. Then in 2002 and again in 2013, researchers compared results of the surgery to a sham version of the operation. There were no differences in outcome between the groups.

A good example of this in oncology is a new class of drugs that are specific for the mutated version of the kinase BRAF (pronounced Bee-Raf). In 2002 the BRAF gene was discovered to be mutated in more than 50 percent of melanomas, as well as in a few other cancers, including up to 10 percent of colon cancers. The most common mutation, V600E, hyperactivates the BRAF kinase activity to induce cancer cells to grow out of control. In 2011 the FDA approved the use of the inhibitor vemurafenib (Zelboraf) in patients with late-stage melanoma. It's a drug that helps patients who previously had few options. Even though it doesn't eradicate the tumors or even hold them back for years, like imatinib does for chronic myeloid leukemias (think Kareem Abdul-Jabbar), it has prolonged patients' lives for several months and led to improvements in symptoms.

Vemurafenib and its cousins work only in patients whose tumors have the BRAF V600E mutation. Unlike the success of BRAF inhibitors in BRAF-mutated melanoma, at the time of this writing BRAF inhibitors have thus far been ineffective in colon cancers with the same BRAF mutation. This was discovered when vemurafenib began to be used off-label in colon cancer patients late in 2011. This was an unexpected result and the use of BRAF inhibitors for BRAF-mutant colon cancers is now on the National Comprehensive Cancer Network's list of therapies that are not recommended for these patients—even though their tumors have the target. Researchers are still working to understand the differences that make BRAF-mutant colon cancers insensitive to BRAF inhibitors. Even when different malignancies exhibit similar mutations, the mutations do not always imply the same tumor biology. In colon cancer, mutations have to be viewed within the context of the colon. "Mutation targeting" in colon cancer is quite distinct (and disappointing) relative to melanoma or chronic myeloid leukemia. Sadly, where you come from matters in tumors, just as it does in people.

In the United States, it's the FDA that evaluates the evidence from clinical trials to determine whether new therapies are safe and effective. In some senses, the FDA is damned if it does and damned if it doesn't. On one side, it gets criticized for delaying the introduction of new therapies by forcing manufacturers to perform time-consuming and expensive clinical trials. On the other side, it also gets criticized if new therapies are prematurely introduced on the market and turn out to have unanticipated risks. The FDA tries to strike a balance to ensure that new drugs are safe and effective. While it may not always get it exactly right, the American public is much better off for the agency's regulation.

The FDA tries to ensure public safety by providing guidance to physicians about what kinds of therapies have proved safe and effective. Manufacturers cannot market drugs for uses other than the ones the FDA has approved. But physicians are free to use new therapies off-label. But for them to do so, the drug has to be approved for *something,* or it wouldn't be on the market in the first place.

Physicians know to think twice about off-label uses (e.g., BRAF-inhibitor use in colon cancer), but off-label use of drugs by physicians has also introduced medical innovations that improve patient care. Bevacizumab (Avastin) is an anti-angiogenesis therapeutic antibody drug approved for palliation of metastatic cancers, but arguably its most successful use is for eye diseases such as wet macular degeneration and diabetic retinopathy. Anti-angiogenesis therapies block the development of new blood vessels. Bevacizumab was developed as an anticancer agent because tumors must promote the development of new blood vessels to supply themselves with the oxygen and nutrients they need to grow. However, wet macular degeneration and diabetic retinopathy is caused by the inappropriate growth of new blood vessels that impair retinal function. This off-label use is acceptable. In fact, although the FDA doesn't officially approve, it tacitly approves by not cracking down.

The FDA has enforcement power to prosecute shysters who sell fraudulent therapies to patients. There is a long history of snake-oil salespeople trying to make a quick buck by selling bogus therapies and false hopes to patients. Since individual patients and physicians rarely have the time or sophistication to critically evaluate the science underlying therapies, countries need agencies like the FDA. With a regulatory regime in which the safety and efficacy of all new therapies are tested in predictable ways, and then evaluated by panels of experts, the general public can have confidence in the safety of our drug system.

In countries that lack an FDA equivalent, snake-oil sales are rampant. Indeed, desperate American patients with incurable diseases are sometimes seduced by hustlers in countries (like Mexico) with poorly regulated medical systems who promise to cure almost anything with sham therapies. These unproven therapies run the gamut from untested truthy ideas that are based on a kernel of truth to outright fraud. The unproven therapies are often marketed to patients with the idea that the FDA or pharmaceutical companies are trying to hide effective therapies from consumers. Unfortunately, desperate patients have a remarkable capacity to suspend disbelief and fall victim to these scams in substantial numbers. If your doctor doesn't have reason to believe a therapy is likely safe and effective, then you should be very wary of that therapy. It's extremely unlikely that an effective new therapy would first be introduced in a private clinic in a third-world country.

Why We Need Clinical Trials

In 1993, back when Bea was diagnosed with metastatic breast cancer, I spoke with her oncologist. He suggested a game plan of chemotherapy to shrink the tumor, followed by a bone marrow transplant. I'd never heard of using a bone marrow transplant to treat breast cancer, not even for breast cancer that had metastasized to the bone marrow, so I polled attending physicians at the Dana-Farber Cancer Institute, where I was doing my oncology rotations. A few were all for the transplant. Others said that using bone marrow transplantation to try to cure metastatic breast cancer was going to go down in history as one of the major fiascos of oncology.

I was fresh out of school, where I'd spent years learning how to do science. My Ph.D. mentor, Phil Majerus, was a master at teaching the scientific method, which meant learning how to set aside wishful thinking to concentrate on the facts. Science is, ultimately, about continually improving your relationship with reality. It's about apprehending the world the way it is, not the way we wish it to be.

But now, I was trying to apply the scientific method to the treatment of my beloved older sister. With cancer progressing to her bones, there weren't many effective treatments available. Chemotherapy would help, but if a bone marrow transplant was a good option, as her doctor claimed, it would offer her much more hope. However, a bone marrow transplant is a harrowing and dangerous procedure for anyone, and even more so for a person with stage IV cancer. Some people die just from the transplant itself. I hoped I would be able to think clearly. That's what all of us have to do as we think about family history, genetic testing, risk management, and, as in Bea's case, evaluating new cancer treatments.

I did some investigation and discovered that a large number of doctors and researchers were enthusiastic about bone marrow transplantation for breast cancer. But the data were weak and based only on a phase II clinical trial. There are four main phases of clinical trials, and each represents an increased level of rigor: Phase 0 measures drug levels in the blood and sometimes in the tumor or other tissues. Phase I tests for drug toxicity and identifies the dose that patients can safely tolerate. Phase II assesses a treatment for possible effectiveness in a limited number of patients. And the most rigorous test of efficacy comes in phase III, when the trials are more stringently controlled and expanded to include many more patients.

Phase II can be a treacherous period. Because of the small

sample sizes and the opportunity for bias, positive phase II results can be misleading and fail to hold up when the trial moves to phase III. These days, when I think about promising new PARP inhibitors or CAR T cell therapies or immune therapies, I remind myself that many of them are still in phase I or phase II testing. Phase III is where the rubber meets the road.

In the case of bone marrow transplants for breast cancer, the positive results of the phase II trial were particularly questionable. Ideally, patients are split into two groups, one that receives the new treatment and a control group that receives the normal standard of care, and then the results are compared. But here, the control group wasn't treated at the same time as the treatment group. Instead, a historical control was used. This means that the researchers didn't do a side-by-side comparison of bone-marrow-transplanted and non-transplanted breast cancer patients to see who had better outcomes. Instead they gave the entire (and small) group of patients the transplant and compared their outcomes to an average picture of how similar patients had fared in the past. The use of historical controls is a notoriously risky path, because patients who are treated at different times can differ in ways that are hard for physicians to identify. Nonetheless, it's often done in phase II trials to reduce costs, with the understanding that if the results are positive, they will have to be confirmed in a phase III trial that investigates more patients and uses randomized side-by-side controls. Basing treatment decisions on phase II trials, especially trials of a punishing and potentially hazardous treatment, is dicey.

One reason that physicians found the idea of bone marrow transplantation compelling, despite the weak evidence, was that the underlying rationale was attractive. Radiation and chemotherapy are often inadequate to cure patients with advanced breast cancer. It was possible that increasing the doses of radiation and chemo would more effectively kill the breast cancer cells, but this strategy is limited by damage to the bone marrow that prevents patients from making enough blood cells to survive. It was logical to wonder if physicians might be able to safely jack up the chemotherapy dose if they transplanted fresh bone marrow into patients after the chemotherapy. Patients could have their cake and eat it too by getting their breast cancer cured by the higher chemotherapy dose while avoiding hematopoietic failure through bone marrow transplantation.

The thought leaders in the transplant area were becoming famous for aggressively pursuing "cures" through transplantation. At the same time, lawyers were hitting the jackpot. The lawsuits against insurance companies that refused to pay for bone marrow transplants (on the grounds that they were still experimental) were settled for enormous sums. In the meantime, patients were suffering from a difficult, risky, and expensive treatment, and insurance companies were increasing their premiums. Doctors and scientists who argued that the therapy should be more fully tested before being used were considered, at best, weak advocates for their patients. At worst, they were called mean and cynical. Even the U.S. government in 1994 made sure its employees had health benefits that included bone marrow transplantation for breast cancer.

Finally, there was a positive phase III study reported by the South African clinician Werner Bezwoda and his research team in 1995. The Bezwoda study gave enormous hope by claiming that 50 percent of the transplanted breast cancer patients had gone into full remission, compared with only 4 percent of those in the control group who hadn't received transplants.

Then four other international phase III trials tried to reproduce Bezwoda's results. They couldn't. In those trials, transplantation did not lead to patients doing better. It turned out that Bezwoda was a fraud. The control groups in the Bezwoda trials weren't even historical. They were imaginary; he made them up.

Why would Bezwoda invent his results? He knew that if

colleagues couldn't reproduce his results at different hospitals, they would ultimately discover his fraud. It appears that he deeply believed that bone marrow transplants would help patients, and he hoped to become famous by being the first to prove it—even if he had to take a shortcut to get there. Sadly, his story is not unique. One of the ways that science and medicine go wrong is under the influence of scientists who are so sure of their pet theories that they cut corners while testing them. They devote themselves to demonstrating the truth of their ideas rather than rigorously testing them.

In the end, the record was corrected by additional randomized phase III trials in which the control subjects were, in fact, real human beings. Bone marrow transplantation was found to be just as ineffective as standard therapy. This is why the most rigorous trials randomly assign patients to treatment categories, often blindly, so that the patient and the physician don't know what treatment group they are in. That way, psychological factors are less likely to influence the outcome of the trial.

The bone marrow transplant story demonstrates why we all have to be careful when we talk and think about targeted treatments for cancer. Cancer is a topic about which people seem to be more prone to deceiving themselves than usual, and sometimes they spread that deceit through the scientific and cultural atmosphere. Confident, hopeful (and competitive) researchers like Werner Bezwoda do it. The doctors who put the scientific method aside when interpreting the phase II trials did it. And researchers and doctors who suggest that new targeted cancer treatments are *without a doubt* going to work are doing it, too. Cancer is just not that simple. If we are going to solve the mysteries in our DNA and if we are going to eventually cure cancer, it all comes down to this: We can't fool ourselves into thinking we know something when we don't. And we have to pursue the truth we *can* know. If we're going to stop cancer, we're going to have to be smart about it. And that means keeping our heads on straight, even when we desperately want to believe that a new therapy or drug is going to be a magic bullet.

Of course, in the early 1990s none of the phase III trials for bone marrow transplantation, whether fraudulent or legitimate, had been published. I had to make a recommendation to Bea based on nothing but a weak phase II trial and interviews with my oncologist teachers. I weighed my hope for a cure against my fear that the transplant could make her illness much worse, much faster. I fell back on my training under Majerus. The data were too weak and the risk to Bea was too great. In fact, I felt that asking a patient to endure a marrow transplant outside a tightly controlled medical trial was almost criminal. Patients receiving unproven therapies should almost *always* be in registered clinical trials so that data can be systematically collected on the effectiveness of the therapy and so that, at the very least, the resulting data can be used to help patients in the future.

I prepared myself to break the news to Bea, and I worried about coming across as cold or unwilling to aggressively pursue a cure. This was not the first or last time I've wished fervently for more data on cancer than is available. If we had more data, especially from people with hereditary cancer syndromes, we could improve therapies so much faster. We could offer more hope of the best kind. We could offer rational hope, based in reality.

In the end, Bea's cancer progressed too fast. I never did have to make a recommendation. Having a transplant turned out not to be an option for her, and soon my attention was focused on helping to make my sister comfortable and mourning her passing. But the lesson I learned from that experience has stuck with me. It's a reason that I worry when I hear chatter and hype about a new treatment or avenue of research. Hype blinds us. It fires our ambition and even our greed. It makes us sloppy.

There's another danger that we all need to fear. Research costs money, and research labs are competing for limited dollars. When one avenue of research, such as research into targeted immunotherapies, gets lots of attention, it can siphon money away from other investigations that are equally promising. For example, there is not enough support for basic scientific investigation of all the newly discovered genes in the genome. Scientists are discovering more and more broken genes in patients with diseases, and few are able to invest the time and resources required to pursue the painstaking research into these genes. But this research is needed to understand the gene products' purposes in the normal cell—so that we can not only develop better treatments for cancer but also identify who's at risk and prevent cancer in the first place.

What about Sequencing the Whole Genome of Your Germline or Tumor?

Come to our cancer treatment center, where we'll sequence your tumor to provide you the best in customized, personalized, targeted medicine.

You have to get your tumor sequenced. Otherwise, how will your doctors know how to treat it?

If I had cancer, I'd get my whole genome sequenced so that doctors could tailor treatment to my DNA.

Ever hear statements like the ones above? There are some out there who suggest that people with cancer need to get the whole genome of their tumor and their germline sequenced in order to receive tailored cancer treatment. As I mentioned earlier, the germline genome is the one you were born with—it's the DNA in all your cells. Your tumor genome is different. It includes all the mutations that occurred in the cancer cells—the somatic mutations that turned them into cancer cells. In other words, your germline genome contains your original blueprints while the tumor genome reflects the modified blueprints after a malignant renovation.

There's value in sequencing certain genes in cancer cells that we know are often mutated, and for which drugs can disable cancer cells by targeting the mutant proteins (imatinib for BCR-ABL, gefitinib for mutant EGFR, and vemurafenib for mutant BRAF). In this way, a certain amount of sequencing in specific genes can help to personalize cancer therapies by identifying what therapies a patient might respond to. However, this idea is increasingly being broadened by the excitement we all feel about the possibility that more genome knowledge will lead to better patient care. Encouraging people to sequence all the genes in tumors, or even the entire genome (not just the genes that encode proteins but all the other DNA sequences between the genes that encode regulatory elements and other things) is an idea. But it's premature to say it's a good idea. We need more data.

In addition to the many drugs that are used to target the aberrations in tumor genomes—whether they come from patients with a genetic predisposition to cancer like the McCoys or not—it's worth recalling that most of the genetic aberrations occur in only the cancer cells, not in germline DNA. For example, BCR-ABL mutations in CML are found only in the cancer cells, so sequencing germline DNA wouldn't tell you if it was present or not. Physicians often sequence a panel of genes in DNA from a patient's cancer cells to look for mutations that are possible targets for existing drugs or that predict the way cancer cells will respond to other therapies. Other kinds of diagnostic tests are also performed on tissue from cancer cells to determine whether they make other kinds of targets, like estrogen receptor and high HER2 levels in breast cancer cells.

Nonetheless, this does not require whole genome sequencing. Targeted sequencing is faster, less expensive, and less likely to return information of uncertain significance that might complicate the treatment plan. There are currently *no* treatments available that require the tumor's whole genome to be sequenced.

Sometimes doctors can start to believe the hype, too. That's why it's so important to remain hopeful about new treatments while not getting carried away. If a doctor or treatment center suggests that you can have "personalized" medicine based on full genome sequencing of your tumor, raise an eyebrow—or both eyebrows. Find out if your insurance company or a research study will cover the cost. If not, ask your doctor for a description of how your treatment would change as a result of this test. If you don't get a clear answer, get a second opinion. In the end, evaluating the state of cancer research depends on the same elements you need when you're researching your family history: tolerating the discomfort of not knowing, honesty, and persistence.

The value of research is best illustrated by taking a look back at some of the women I've written about in this book. In the 1950s, 1980s, and early 1990s, when Rosalind Franklin, Gilda Radner, and Bea were treated for their cancers, we had no knowledge of genes called BRCA1 or BRCA2. Even when these mutant genes were discovered in patients with ovarian and breast cancers in the mid-1990s, we thought there was no use in testing women for them. At the time, we didn't know of any strategies or therapies that would change outcomes for patients with these mutations. But in 2006, Bea's daughter turned eighteen. She was able to get tested for a BRCA mutation and take action to avoid an early death like her mother's. Other people with mutations in VHL, RET, and other MLH1 genes are doing the same. Not a single one of them would be able to claim this power if it weren't for research, even with all its sand traps, potholes, and speed bumps.

Chapter Eight

Science Is a Group Project:
Data Points and You

IT'S AN UNSEASONABLY WARM JUNE 14 in the Upper Midwest, and on this Flag Day my family is taking advantage of the good weather to throw a birthday party for Grammy, who is turning ninety. It's a pretty good excuse for a family reunion. Family members have traveled from around the globe to meet at Grammy's assisted-living center in Ann Arbor for a celebratory concert played by an ensemble formed by my brothers, nieces, and nephews.

But this is more than a family reunion. I've always wanted to research BRCA mutations. To do that, I wanted research material from a family of BRCA mutants.

As it turns out, I happen to know of one.

A genetic counselor stands up in front of the gaggle of family members to deliver a consent speech. After we've signed waivers and release forms, the beer and lemonade begin to flow as a nurse and dermatologist stand at the ready. One by one, Grammy, my brothers, sisters-in-law, uncle, aunt, nieces, and nephews have their blood drawn by the nurse. The dermatologist, a longtime friend, takes samples of the skin on their arms and sews things up with a stitch or two.

Bea's daughter has made a special trip home from Peace Corps service in Ukraine to attend Grammy's party. We already know her BRCA1 mutation status, so we grant her a compassionate exemption from yet another of the blood draws she hates so much. Bea's son says he'll do anything he can to help with research. (A few years later, Bea's son will unofficially change his middle name from Ross to Rosenblum, to honor the Jewish origins of his maternal line.)

The party migrates to our house, where Grammy poses with her nine grandchildren for a photo. Grammy sometimes gets confused and tells people that she has twenty-nine grandchildren. It's another case of inaccurate family history reporting, but we'll make sure the facts are straight for the data collectors. Grammy's surviving ninety-something friends have traveled from Kalamazoo with their caretakers to help celebrate. Room is made for walkers and wheelchairs. Presents are exchanged all around, opened by the wrong ninety-year-olds, and a happy confusion reigns. Those of us in middle age have the usual discussion about how teenagers are like terrorists, willing to strike with deft precision at their family's weakest spots.

Bea's daughter's innocent voice chimes in. "I had no idea," she says.

"I know," I say. "But parents understand. Teenagers are supposed to be terrible."

She instantly corrects me. "No, I mean I had no idea that everyone expects teenagers to misbehave. If I'd known that it was an option when I was a teenager, I would have been a lot worse!" Her father and stepmother, standing close by, raise their brows ever so slightly.

Uncle Manny talks to anyone who's willing to listen about the experiments that might be done with our blood and skin samples.

As a man of science, he understands that genetics is, essentially, the study of families, and that the goal of most genetic researchers is to collect material from several members of the same family. My lab will bank the samples from the BRCA1 mutants and the non-mutants. We and others can use these samples to better understand how BRCA1 mutations lead to cancer. While Manny is exulting, I'm reveling in the fact I've finally put my own skin (the skin biopsies included my own) in the game for BRCA research.

The family's enthusiasm is not dampened when I explain that although my lab is going to use their donations to research the BRCA1 gene, it's always possible that the research won't come up with anything. Research goes down a lot of blind alleys. Even if research on the family's samples turns up useful information, and even if that information could potentially help family members manage their medical decisions, the family won't be told about it. Before their samples are used for research, they will be so thoroughly de-identified that the samples will only have the medical information of the individual linked to the sample. I know which sample corresponds to which family member because I happen to know them all, and the relevant parts of their medical history. However, sample de-identification will prevent anyone else from linking samples or data to any individual. Furthermore, before research results are applied to the real world, they need to be verified in a clinical lab that is regulated by the government for technical accuracy. My family is not going to get any direct benefit or knowledge from the research, no matter what. But they all want to be part of the solution to the problem of cancer, even if their contribution is unacknowledged or minute. I felt proud to be associated with all of them that day, mutants and nonmutants alike.

At this point you might ask, *What about you, Theo? Isn't it a conflict of interest to research your family? Will you learn anything about yourself?*

To eliminate a conflict of interest, I took no active part in either the consent process or the process of getting the research approved by an institutional review board, an independent ethics panel that reviews investigations that involve human subjects.

I did learn something about myself, though. I learned from the genome sequences that the Ross/Rosenblums have a so-called mutation in a gene called CBP. This mutation, based on a few reports in the literature, is supposed to cause Rubinstein-Taybi syndrome, a devastating childhood developmental disorder that can lead to leukemia, lymphoma, and other cancers. But none of us has the disease. After finding CBP in the family samples, I went through phases when I'd stare at family photos, trying to identify any physical features that could suggest a mild form of the disease. Only by squinting and revving my notorious imagination was I able to convince myself that we might have the unusual faces, hands, and feet that are hallmarks of the Rubinstein-Taybi syndrome. No, there is no sign that any of us are afflicted with the syndrome.

This discovery—that a CBP "mutation" can be present in a family that is free of Rubinstein-Taybi syndrome—shows why family gene studies are so valuable. Some of the research studies that show links between mutations and diseases are based on very small sample sizes. New research with more subjects is casting some of those supposedly harmful mutations in a different light. Some of them are less ominous than we previously thought, or even neutral. This situation goes beyond cancer. Here in our lab we recently found that a large number of our cancer genetics patients have a mutation that supposedly causes pancreatitis in many of its carriers. But none of the patients have been diagnosed with pancreatitis or have a history of symptoms that could reflect pancreatitis. It's possible that this "mutation" has been given an undeservedly bad reputation. It may just be a normal genetic variant. The same may be true for the CBP mutation we found. As an article in *Science Translational Medicine* in 2011 concluded, "We found an unexpectedly high proportion (27 percent) of literature-annotated disease mutations that were incorrect, incomplete or common polymorphisms. Differentiation of common polymorphisms from disease mutations requires genotyping a large number of unaffected individuals." Translation: Too much is made of research on very small numbers of people. We need more research and more research subjects. This has crucial implications for people who might make life-changing decisions based on what is known about mutations.

The good news is that conclusions based on limited numbers of people are hypotheses; they don't immediately influence clinical care. For example, the CBP "mutation" that we found in our family was based on just a few patients in a few published reports. Few doctors would use that kind of data to make medical recommendations in the clinic. The patient numbers were too small. The data didn't stop me from squinting and searching for symptoms—but this is where training comes in handy. Working to continuously improve our connection to reality is a process all physicians include in their practice of medicine. It also shows how important participation in research is—we need numbers to make solid conclusions.

I learned a few more things from my family's contributions, though not about my genes. Until the family reunion, I didn't study the biology of BRCA genes in my lab, and my research didn't use human samples. My family's generous participation helped me become the human geneticist I wanted to be. It wasn't just that I now had samples to work with. As I observed and worked through the process of institutional review board approval, consent, sample collection, storage, and the first few experiments, I received an education in human subjects research. I'm grateful to Grammy and the rest of my family for giving me that opportunity. I learned that getting institutional review board approval of a project is not as hard and bureaucratic as it seems; that human sample collection can be either simple or fraught with mix-ups; that storage is something that needs to be safeguarded and ensured by keeping duplicate samples and data at different institutions; and that the people you work with have to be organized and of high integrity—they need to admit when they've mixed things up. We made some mistakes, but research is like everything else: If you are honest about your errors, you get valuable feedback that helps you improve the process. Purposeful practice is the best way to learn. And having my family available to use for purposeful practice was like having a mannequin available for CPR practice.

Usually it's hard to get material from such a big family to study (there are exceptions that I'll describe in moment), but we did it. The Ross/Rosenblums provided data and samples from three generations, and the samples are being used together with material from other patients to learn more about what causes cancer to appear in some people with BRCA gene mutations but not in others. A person with a BRCA1 mutation has a 50 to 87 percent chance of getting breast cancer before age eighty. Those sound like high-risk numbers, and they are, but they represent a significant spread. If we could understand what causes the difference in risk, we could be more precise in our recommendations for preventive surgeries versus surveillance. This kind of question can't be answered without crowdsourcing patient data.

A family like mine might be able to help. We know that Grammy has a BRCA1 mutation, but why did she avoid breast cancer until she was seventy-three years old, whereas Bea developed a much more aggressive cancer at age thirty-five? It helps researchers to know the specifics of the family history: To our knowledge, Grammy's brothers and sisters had no early-onset cancers. And Grammy's cancer was estrogen receptor positive, a sign that her cancer might not have been BRCA1-related. (Tumors with BRCA1 mutations are frequently estrogen receptor negative.) Scientists believe there are modifier mutations that interact with BRCA1 and BRCA2 to alter the risk of cancer in some people. What if, for example, the "mutant" CBP gene in our family worked together with a broken BRCA1 to cause Bea's death? Or what if Grumpy's family contributed a different mutation that might have had the same effect? That's one reason I asked Uncle Manny, Grumpy's brother, to join us and donate samples from my paternal line.

If we're going to learn how to prevent, treat, and cure cancer, we need more data points like the ones my family provided. We need more research groups to have the resources and support to launch studies of families, and more families who will share their data. If we could stitch together everyone's stories, they would mean so much more. The data in aggregate will teach us how to manage the risks, how to treat the diseases, how to save lives.

Privacy, Consent, and Good Data-Sharing

At a desk in a laboratory that manages the UT Southwestern Cancer Center's research repository, a staff member receives an incoming shipment of human tissue samples. Each sample is labeled with the patient's identifying information (name, date of birth, medical record number). Before any of these samples can be put into this research repository, the staff member must assign each sample a specific research number that is linked to the donor's medical record number. This research number can be used only by the repository to obtain updated health history from the patient's doctor. The staff member permanently destroys the sample's label, which might have other identifying information, including name, date of birth, contact information, any geographical information that is smaller than a state, social security number, medical record number, and any other piece of information that is unique to that person. However, the clinical data relevant to the study, such as cancer history, other health history, and age, stay with the sample.

This is de-identification at work; this process is used to preserve patient privacy. The blood, tissue, or tumor sample is linked to a patient's story but the name is removed and replaced with a number. When there is new clinical data, only the patient's health-care team can update the sample information by communicating with the lab. (The patient's identifying information remains in the medical record that is linked to the sample.)

Our lab has material from four generations of a family whose members have unusually high rates of kidney cancers and hemangioblastomas, a type of brain cancer. We call them the "mystery kidney cancer family" because they definitely have a familial cancer syndrome, but as of yet, no clinical test has diagnosed the genetic cause. There is another good reason to call them the "mystery family." None of the basic science researchers, the ones who spin the blood samples through centrifuges and extract the DNA for analysis, have met any of the family members. They know what kind of cancers the family members have had, their ages, and other health data. But the people in the lab who are key to figuring out what's wrong in this family's gene pool do not know any of the personal identifiers. And the family knows that although its samples are being used to conduct research, we cannot pass our research results back to them—not even if we find the mutation that causes their cancers. Despite this, the family is all in. So is their doctor. All parties understand that there is a line between the early basic research and the patients, and this line is bright and red.

This de-identification and separation during basic research comes before any clinical research takes place. It's the kind of research that was carried out in 1951, when the first cancer cell line to grow indefinitely in a culture dish (many tumor cells were grown transiently in culture prior to this), known as HeLa, was cultured from Henrietta Lacks, a woman with cervical cancer. Per the usual practice at that time, the cells were taken from Lacks's surgical specimen without her knowledge. The standards for consent have evolved over time and continue to evolve today: The ethical standards in the 1970s, or even in the 1990s, were not as good as they are today. Modern research rules are different. They require that donors sign detailed consent forms and that, when promised, de-identification is performed prior to the sample's use in basic research. We've come a long way in the protection of patients' privacy. It's an entirely new era, with better safeguards and protections.

In 2013, a controversy erupted when the journal *Science* published an article claiming that if a lab sequences a person's whole genome, the data can be used to identify the person—even if the person's name isn't attached. This would mean that a person could get wind of his or her research-grade results, but those results could be wrong. Or someone could discover they have a mutation for an incurable, untreatable disease like Alzheimer's or Huntington's, even if they didn't want to have that knowledge. But this claim was based on a study that didn't thoroughly de-identify the samples. The *Science* article showed that the sample could be re-identified *only* if the lab provides other telltale information about the subject, such as zip code and birthday. But standard de-identification procedures don't allow these details to appear with samples, so the risk of privacy invasion or unwanted identification is low.

An interesting twist in the *Science* story is that when participants in the Personal Genome Project, a sequencing project led by Dr. George Church of Harvard University, were informed there was a possibility that they could be identified from their DNA sequence and the possible consequences were explained (they even had to take a test to prove they understood), few people dropped out of the study. It turns out that for many people, privacy wasn't as important as what could be gained by using the data to understand and treat disease. Privacy isn't everything! In fact, there is increasing evidence that people are becoming less and less concerned about privacy with the ascent of social media.

Let's Build Data-Sharing Plans
for Cancer Genetics

What happens when two clinical testing labs interpret one patient's genetic data in different ways? As I write this book, we've been working with a woman who developed breast cancer at the age of thirty-three. We discovered that she has a mutation in a gene, called CHEK2, which predisposes her to breast, colon, and other cancers. Now the woman's little sister has come to see us for genetic counseling. She's tested negative for the CHEK2 mutation that her big sister has, the one that's known to increase cancer risk. But something unusual has popped up: She has a *different* mutation in the CHEK2 gene, one that we haven't seen very often. Remember, everyone has two copies of each gene, one from each parent. She's inherited a different mutation from her parents than her older sister did. The first testing lab tentatively concluded that the younger sister's mutation is harmful, too. Having had little experience with this particular mutation, we weren't so sure. We sent her information to a second lab, which concluded that her CHEK2 mutation isn't so bad after all—just a harmless variant. The second lab had accumulated more data on the mutation and was able to come to a more confident conclusion.

This kind of disagreement and uncertainty between genetic testing labs is fairly rare, but it's going to become more common. New sequencing tools and increased testing will dig up more and more genetic variants. Often we won't know whether these variants are harmful or whether they are simply alternate but perfectly valid genetic sequences—like the spellings of "check" and "cheque," different letters that mean the same thing. Our ability to sequence patients' DNA is outstripping our ability to interpret the information. From a single person's genome, we can get a terabyte of data, almost three billion base pairs of sequence. We just don't know what most of that data mean. With each single gene that is sequenced, we have to ask ourselves these questions:

Is this sequence normal?

If not, does this sequence lead to a higher or a lower risk for the patient?

Does this sequence work in combination with other genes to alter health outcomes?

One way to address this problem is to discourage clinical labs from thinking they own the data associated with patients' test results. A prime example is the lack of access to a database of sequences of the BRCA1 and BRCA2 genes from hundreds of thousands patients sequenced by Myriad Genetics, a major testing lab. What if it had been required through the FDA approval process that Myriad Genetics share its insurance-funded test results since 1996? We'd all know a lot more about the normal and cancer-causing BRCA1 and BRCA2 variants. We need to encourage labs to share their data with one another. Competition in some situations is productive, but in the case of seeking meaning in our genomes, it's costly and counterproductive. Beyond the human tendency toward competition, there are also policy, legal, and information technology hurdles that make data sharing a challenge. Still, data sharing among commercial as well as research laboratories is key and must be facilitated. Cancer research should be a group project. The data should be community property so that doctors can ultimately use that data to make the best recommendations for their patients.

What if the two companies could have compared the younger sister's CHEK2 mutation to a database that contains a lot more data than any single lab's database? Both labs could have seen that the younger sister's DNA likely had a benign sequence found in people without an elevated cancer risk. The first lab wouldn't have called it "likely harmful," and she wouldn't have considered taking unnecessary steps to manage a miscalculated risk.

My own lab just reported on our analyses of the sequences of the whole genomes of 258 patients from our cancer genetics clinic. We discovered new mutations that we speculate work in tandem with well-known mutations, such as those that cause Lynch syndrome or BRCA mutations, to cause cancer. Recall that we and others are working to identify new gene sequences that could explain why some patients with BRCA mutations have cancer by the time they are thirty-five (Bea) and others with the same mutations are cancer-free during their entire lifetime. These new mutations don't fully explain the 50 to 87 percent risk spread in all of our BRCA1 mutant patients, but we now have hypotheses. We need more data from more patients to validate and test our findings. To begin to address this, we have deposited the data in a public database run by the National Institutes of Health (NIH), known as database of Genotypes and Phenotypes (dbGaP), so that it will be available for scientists to see, to reinterpret, to compare with their data, and to come up with their own hypotheses. Putting the data into dbGaP was a large effort. We needed to upload not only massive amounts of sequence data to the NIH database, but also each of the subject's personal and family medical histories, which was labor-intensive, detailed, and very expensive. If laboratories shared their data with public databases—like dbGaP for research-grade data and the other NIH databases such as ClinVar and the Genetic Testing Registry for clinical-grade data—we'd know more, faster, about the impact the sequences have on health.

A public database won't be maximally helpful unless we can take the data and connect it to patient and family health histories. DNA alone simply isn't enough. We need to link the genetic information to accurate family health information: whether they've developed cancer or heart disease or Alzheimer's; whether they've taken risk-management measures; whether they've been exposed to known carcinogens (like cigarette smoke); and what their medical outcomes have been. Around the world, other countries are beginning to set up their own data banks. In 2006, the U.K. Biobank began to recruit five hundred thousand adults ages forty to sixty-nine for a twenty-five-year study. Scientists there are collecting blood and urine samples, getting clinical information through questionnaires, and taking physical measurements. In essence, they're logging stories so that they can make links between genes, lifestyles, and health. They are targeting people in midlife, because they are the ones most likely to have first diagnoses of common diseases like cancer, heart disease, stroke, diabetes, and dementia. The dbGaP, which the NIH established in 2007, has collected research data from more than five hundred studies at the time of this writing. It's a good model, and one that is growing. Iceland has had a database with genetic, lifestyle, and health information since 1996. As I write, President Barack Obama is calling for the collection of one million sequenced genomes. We are moving in the right direction, but we need public pressure on regulatory agencies, insurance companies, and health-care providers around the world to keep these projects alive.

What Families Can Do to Accelerate Cancer Research

Patients with hereditary predispositions to cancer (or any disease) should never have to worry that their identifying information will be made available to the public. Fortunately, maintaining genetic privacy and participation in research are not mutually exclusive. We are all one big human family, and the more we know about our inherited predispositions toward cancer, the less that patients will have to make clinical decisions in the dark. Already, families like mine are beginning to participate in research so that all of us can take advantage of the power in their blood.

I'll conclude by telling you about another family that is sharing its stories so that the next generation can thrive. It's an ideal family for research. To limit the variables that can affect health, members of this family would need to eat similarly, live in the same area, and never smoke or drink. They would live in the same way for several generations and keep detailed records of their health and other personal characteristics. Their records would be accurate. They would intermarry to reduce genetic diversity within the community. There would be little confusion about paternity. It sounds like a luxury colony of laboratory mice, but it's not. It's a really big human family. It's the Mormons.

Mormons are not the only group of people who are genetically distinct. In the United States, there are the Amish and the Mennonites; in Quebec, the French Canadians. Iceland, where many family histories reach back a thousand years, has created genetic family trees in great detail. But the number of Mormons who make themselves available for genetic study is unprecedented.

Between the 1840s and 1890s, a subgroup of Mormons practiced polygamy for a few generations. Some men fathered as many as fifty children with multiple wives; the sons in turn also had large numbers of children. Today, thousands of Mormon families are descended from this group, which means that the genes of a small number of men have been amplified and entrenched in the Mormon genetic landscape. Tracing those genes through the branches of the family can teach us a lot about how specific traits move through generations.

The Mormons have also given the scientific community a culture that is conducive to genetic discovery. The Mormon Church, which considers family history sacred information, has made it easy to collect family histories. Since 1836, the church has invested much time and resources bringing records together in a family history library that is located in downtown Salt Lake City. It's the largest collection of family histories in the world.

By the mid-twentieth century, geneticists realized the Mormons owned a research treasure chest. Mark Skolnick, Ph.D., a professor and leader of genetics at the University of Utah, and his team used the library to scour the records of people who were born, died, or married in Utah. He also looked at the Utah cancer registry, which has documented all cancers in the state since 1966. By putting the two together, Skolnick identified when cancer was running in families. The Utah cancer registry and the Mormon family records library have a million or so records in common! Skolnick led a team of researchers that, by culling information from this registry and studying the genetics of families with increased cancer incidences, eventually discovered cancer-predisposing BRCA1 mutations. (He and his colleagues built their work on Mary-Claire King's observation that a familial breast cancer syndrome was associated with changes in a particular chromosome.)

The Mormons' lifestyle helps, too. They have an average of eight children (it's hard to perform genetic research on families with only one child). They are ethnically homogenous when compared with the rest of the population—most are of Scandinavian descent. And they don't smoke or drink. All this makes it easier to separate genetic influence on health from lifestyle factors.

Mormon families invite researchers from the Huntsman Cancer Institute, a research facility affiliated with the University of Utah, to their family reunions, where members eagerly contribute samples for research. These participating families are true research partners. They also have a strong sense of community and citizenship that makes them want to contribute to scientific knowledge, even if that knowledge doesn't directly help them or their own family. With grace and efficiency, these Mormon families have advanced the study of genetics. More discoveries of disease-causing mutations have occurred in Utah than anywhere else, including mutations in BRCA1 and BRCA2, APC (the familial adenomatous polyposis colon cancer gene), and CDKN2A (known as the "melanoma gene").

Certainly, the genetic value of my family pales to that of the Mormons. We're not that large. We have few biological children. We are geographically dispersed, and we can't boast the same kind of clean living as the Mormons. Still, that shouldn't stop us or other families from participating in research. There are things that the Ross/Rosenblums and the Mormons have in common that are useful for researchers. We're available, open to change, communicative with one another and our doctors, and tolerant of medical uncertainty—and we're always interesting. If you've got an inherited cancer syndrome, ask your genetic counselor about donating samples for research. If your family members are willing, ask the counselor if *all* of you can donate samples. There might be a study that can use your samples right away, or perhaps the clinic or lab can de-identify and store your samples for future use.

When I learned about my BRCA1 mutation, I was sitting in my office on a wintry day in Michigan, waiting for news that would change my life. In the final days of writing this book, I've been working from my new office in Dallas, where my lab is studying the genetic material from cancer-prone families, hoping to lay a foundation for better prevention and treatments of inherited cancers. My new office looks a lot like the one I had in Michigan. There's a round table in the center, and the shelves are decorated with books and photos of patients, special colleagues, and family. But many things are not the same.

Life really has changed. Instead of facing a 50 to 87 percent chance of developing breast cancer in my lifetime, my risk has plummeted to the level of an average woman's—and possibly lower. I no longer have to spend mental energy pushing aside my worries about cancer. I don't have to fear for my family the way I used to. In the lab and clinic, I'm doing the work I've always wanted to do. Plus, it's springtime here in Texas. The air is warm, the azaleas are blooming, and the sky is big and blue. I smile, knowing that a few miles down the road, Grammy—now age ninety-four—is sitting on the patio of her assisted-living facility, sunbathing and enjoying the company of her boyfriend. I've been reading the pages of this manuscript to Grammy, a little at a time.

Instead of waiting nervously for a call, the way I did that day in Michigan, I pick up the phone myself. First I call my brothers, and then I send an email to Uncle Manny. I explain to each of them that I've written a book about cancer genetics and family—and that *their* genes and *their* stories are woven into its pages. Do I have their permission to share our family's experience? Their answers are resoundingly positive. They hope the book will somehow make its way to my mother's side of the family, so that our unknown relatives can learn about their cancer risk and then protect themselves. Uncle Manny is excited about spreading the news beyond our blood kin. "How wonderful," he writes, "to advance public knowledge about cancer genetics through our family."

The Ross/Rosenblums understand something that I've said throughout this book: Knowing about a cancer mutation gives you power. It gives you options and lets *you* make decisions before cancer makes them for you. If we expand the amount of data available to scientists and physicians, and fund more cancer research, the future will be better for all of us. We could treat cancer more precisely. Better still, we could prevent it more often. We're all members of the same human family. By sharing our information with one another, we make better health available to all of our "relatives" in the widest sense, and to the generations that follow.

ACKNOWLEDGMENTS

I am deeply indebted to the patients and their families who have shared their lives and stories with me in St. Louis, Boston, Ann Arbor, and Dallas. They have taught me more and contributed more to this book's content than the best textbooks.

In addition to soulful gratitude to my husband, Sean Morrison, as the senior "Ideal Reader" and Director of the book's Support Staff, there were the dear friends who assisted me in this project as "ideal readers" or "ideal supporters." In particular I'd like to thank: the Bostonians, Janet Jacobs and Susanne Dowdall; the Ohioan, Heather Hampel; and the Dallasites, Lucy and Henry Billingsley, and Caren and Pete Kline.

I am grateful to colleagues, especially the nurses and counselors I've had the opportunity to work with and learn from. Most relevant to this book are our genetic counselors here at UT Southwestern Medical Center: Linda Robinson, Megan Frone, Caitlin Mauer, Sara Pirzadeh-Miller, Lesli Kiedrowski, Jillian Huang, and Jacqueline Mersch. One of my motivations to write this book was to learn more about genetics so that I could keep up with them. I also thank Drs. Judy Garber, Charis Eng, and Bob Nussbaum for their confidence in this project before it was finished.

I am grateful to my agent, Ike Williams, for taking me in, understanding how driven I was to write this book, and showing me the literary ropes. Sadly, Ike's beloved wife, Noa, succumbed to lung cancer during our work together. I am grateful to Katherine Flynn for enthusiastically partnering with Ike so that there was always somebody who could answer my questions.

Thanks to my editors: Leigh Ann Hirschman, Brittney Ross, and Caroline Sutton. Leigh Ann helped me fit the pieces of this story into their right places. She told me the bitter truth when favorite passages needed to be sacrificed and kept the faith in this project. Brittney, my first editor at Penguin Random House, edited with precision; pointed out blind spots; and guided with care, compassion, humor, rapid communication, and, when necessary, silence. Caroline's continuous enthusiasm and wisdom rounded out the team.

I also thank Tony Ross for the clarity of his viewpoint. He provided the working title for this book, *Who's Your Daddy*. This was a fun working title and a concise way of expressing the book's theme. One mention of *Who's Your Daddy* led to instant recognition and interest . . . except from the publisher. The experienced and talented team at Penguin Random House (again led by Caroline Sutton) helped me maintain appropriate boundaries.

I'm grateful to all of the researchers who have taken the field of cancer genetics from that small world pioneered by Drs. Lynch, Li, and Fraumeni in the 1960s to what it is now. I apologize to the members of that pioneering community whose work was not specifically cited. If this were a scientific paper, the citations would have been longer than the book.

Finally, I want to acknowledge the large community of current and future cancer-gene-mutation carriers for their courage and willingness to share with the world their own genetic heritage so we can continue to grow the tree of genetic knowledge and change the future.

APPENDIX 1

Inherited Cancer Syndromes

HEREDITARY BREAST CANCER SYNDROMES

Hereditary Breast and Ovarian Cancer Syndrome (HBOC)

ASSOCIATED GENES: BRCA1 and BRCA2

ASSOCIATED CANCERS: breast cancer, ovarian cancer, male breast cancer, prostate cancer, pancreatic cancer, colon cancer, gastric cancer, and melanoma. BRCA2 gene mutations are also associated with Fanconi anemia, a cancer syndrome described on page 216.

Patterns that suggest HBOC include:

* Breast cancer diagnosed before age forty-five
* Ovarian cancer at any age
* Personal or family history of male breast cancer
* Triple-negative breast cancer diagnosed at or under age sixty
* Personal history of pancreatic or prostate cancer *and* two or more family members with breast, ovarian, prostate, or pancreatic cancer
* Breast cancer diagnosed at or under age fifty *and* one other family member with breast cancer

- Breast cancer at any age *and*:
  - One family member with breast cancer at or under age fifty or ovarian cancer at any age
  - Two or more family members with breast cancer, pancreatic cancer, or prostate cancer
  - Ashkenazi Jewish ancestry

Li-Fraumeni Syndrome

ASSOCIATED GENE: TP53

ASSOCIATED CANCERS: breast cancer, soft-tissue sarcoma, osteosarcoma, brain tumors (primarily choroid plexus carcinoma and glioblastoma), colon cancer, pancreas cancer, prostate cancer, skin cancer, adrenocortical carcinoma, hematological malignancies (primarily leukemia), and ovarian tumors

People with Li-Fraumeni syndrome are radiosensitive and are at increased risk for cancers when exposed to extraneous radiation. Patterns that suggest Li-Fraumeni syndrome include:

- Breast cancer at or before age thirty-five
- Personal or family history of the cancers associated with Li-Fraumeni syndrome (listed above), particularly if those cancers occurred at an early age

ATM

ASSOCIATED CANCERS: breast cancer and pancreatic cancer. Possibly prostate cancer, melanoma, oral and throat cancers, endometrial cancer, and hematological malignancies

Most of the information here pertains to ATM with one inherited gene mutation, known as a heterozygous mutation. People with two ATM gene mutations (homozygous mutations) will develop a rare serious genetic condition called ataxia telangiectasia. This condition typically develops in childhood with motor problems, immunodeficiency, and increased lifetime risks for malignancies. People who have homozygous ATM mutations are sensitive to radiation and experience increased malignancy risks with radiation exposure. (It is not yet clear if people with heterozygous ATM gene mutations are sensitive to radiation exposure.)

There are currently no established patterns that suggest ATM gene mutations. People with a personal or family history of early-onset breast cancer should consider ATM testing as part of a testing panel for hereditary cancer predisposition. People with a personal or family history of ataxia telangiectasia syndrome should also consider ATM gene testing.

BARD1, BRIP1, MRE11A, RAD50, RAD51C, RAD51D

ASSOCIATED CANCERS: breast cancer and possibly ovarian cancer. BRIP1 and RAD51C are also associated with Fanconi anemia syndrome (see page 216).

There are currently no established patterns that suggest BARD1, BRIP1, MRE11A, RAD50, RAD51C, or RAD51D. People with a personal or family history of early-onset or familial breast and/or ovarian cancer should consider testing of these genes as part of a hereditary-cancer-predisposition gene panel.

CHEK2

ASSOCIATED CANCERS: breast cancer, colon cancer, and prostate cancer; possibly ovarian cancer, thyroid cancer, and renal cancer

There are currently no established testing criteria for CHEK2 gene mutations. People with personal and/or family history of breast cancer, particularly if colon cancer is present, should consider testing for this gene as part of a hereditary-cancer-predisposition gene panel. CHEK2 gene mutations can also predispose to later-onset breast cancers.

NBN

ASSOCIATED CANCERS: breast cancer and possibly ovarian cancer

The information here pertains to individuals with only one NBN mutation. People with two NBN mutations will develop a serious genetic condition called Nijmegen breakage syndrome, which is characterized by small stature and microcephaly, cognitive and developmental disabilities, and increased malignancy risks.

There are currently no established testing criteria for NBN gene mutations. People with early-onset or familial breast and/or ovarian cancer should consider testing of this gene as part of a hereditary-cancer-predisposition gene panel.

PALB2

ASSOCIATED CANCERS: breast cancer, pancreatic cancer, and possibly ovarian cancer

PALB2 mutations are also associated with Fanconi anemia syndrome (see page 216).

There are currently no established testing criteria for PALB2. Individuals with a personal and/or family history of breast and/or pancreatic cancer, particularly early-onset, should consider testing for this gene as part of a hereditary-cancer-predisposition gene panel.

Cowden Syndrome

ASSOCIATED GENE: PTEN

ASSOCIATED CANCERS: breast cancer, thyroid cancer (particularly follicular-type thyroid cancer), endometrial cancer, colon cancer, and renal cancer

Individuals with Cowden syndrome also may develop many other benign clinical findings including thyroid nodules and goiter, skin findings, and uterine fibroids. PTEN gene mutations are also associated with Bannayan-Riley-Ruvalcaba syndrome (BRRS) and Proteus syndrome—genetic syndromes that are associated with multiple clinical findings including intestinal polyps and birth defects.

Patterns that suggest Cowden syndrome include:

- Personal or family history of BRRS or Proteus syndrome
- Autism and macrocephaly (large head circumference: 58 centimeters in women or 60 centimeters in men)
- Individuals with skin features associated with Cowden syndrome
- Lhermitte-Duclos disease—a brain finding that can be seen in Cowden syndrome
- Two or more major criteria (see below; one must be macrocephaly)
- Three major criteria (without macrocephaly)
- One major and three or more minor criteria
- Four or more minor criteria

Major Criteria	Minor Criteria
· Breast cancer	· Autism spectrum disorder
· Uterine cancer	· Colon cancer
· Follicular thyroid cancer	· Three or more esophageal glycogenic acanthoses
· Multiple GI hamartomas or ganglioneuromas	· Lipomas
· Macrocephaly	· Intellectual disability
· Macular pigmentation of the glans penis	· Papillary or follicular variant of papillary thyroid cancer
· Skin findings, including trichilemmomas, palmoplantar keratoses, oral papillomas, or multiple facial skin papules	· Thyroid structural lesions (e.g., adenoma, nodule, goiter)
	· Renal cell carcinoma
	· Single GI hamartoma or ganglioneuroma
	· Testicular lipomatosis
	· Vascular anomalies such as arteriovenous malformations or hemangiomas

HEREDITARY COLORECTAL CANCER SYNDROMES

Familial Adenomatous Polyposis (FAP)

ASSOCIATED GENE: APC

ASSOCIATED CANCERS: polyposis, colon cancer, duodenal cancer, gastric cancer, small bowel cancer, pancreatic cancer, thyroid cancer, central nervous system cancer, desmoid tumor (a benign, fibrous tumor that can develop anywhere in the body), and hepatoblastoma under age five

Patterns that suggest FAP include:

- More than ten adenomatous (precancerous type) colon polyps
- A desmoid tumor at any age
- Hepatoblastoma
- Family history of polyposis or cancer may not be observed, as 20 to 25 percent of FAP is the result of a new genetic mutation affecting only one person in the family

Hereditary Diffuse Gastric Cancer (HDGC)

ASSOCIATED GENE: CDH1

ASSOCIATED CANCERS: diffuse gastric cancer and lobular breast cancer; possibly colorectal cancer

Patterns that suggest HDGC include:

- Two gastric cancer cases in the family with one family member diagnosed under age fifty
- Three first- or second-degree relatives with gastric cancer at any age
- Diffuse gastric cancer diagnosed under age forty
- Diffuse gastric cancer and lobular breast cancer in the same person
- Personal and/or family history of diffuse gastric cancer and lobular breast cancer with at least one case diagnosed before age fifty

Lynch Syndrome (also called Hereditary Non-Polyposis Colon Cancer Syndrome, or HNPCC)

ASSOCIATED GENES: MLH1, MSH2, MSH6, PMS2, and EPCAM

ASSOCIATED CANCERS: colon cancer, endometrial cancer, ovarian cancer, gastric and small bowel cancer, central nervous system cancer, pancreatic cancer, bladder/ureter cancer, renal cancer, sebaceous skin and neoplasms; possibly breast cancer

Patterns that suggest Lynch syndrome include:

- Any colorectal or endometrial cancer with abnormal immunohistochemical (IHC) analysis for the mismatch repair (MMR) proteins for Lynch syndrome. IHC analysis is a test performed on the tumor where the tumor is "stained" for the proteins made by the Lynch syndrome genes. If the IHC test is normal (i.e., the proteins stain positive), it suggests that the Lynch syndrome genes are working properly to produce their proteins. If the IHC test is abnormal (i.e., the stain is missing), it suggests that those proteins may not be getting produced correctly and that the genes could not be working properly, suggesting a diagnosis of Lynch syndrome.

- Colorectal cancer with microsatellite-high (MSI-H) histology diagnosed in a patient who is less than sixty years of age (when the Lynch syndrome genes are not working properly, multiple tiny "mismatch" errors can be made in the unstable DNA and lead to many repeats within the DNA sequence that can be measured in the tumor; this is strongly suggestive that that person has Lynch syndrome)

- Colorectal cancer, ovarian cancer, or uterine cancer diagnosed under the age of fifty

- Two or more cancers that are associated with Lynch syndrome

- Colorectal cancer diagnosed in a first-degree relative with a

Lynch syndrome–related tumor diagnosed before the age of fifty

- Colorectal cancer diagnosed in two or more first- or second-degree relatives with a Lynch syndrome–associated tumor, at any age

Multiple Adenomatous Polyposis (MAP)

ASSOCIATED GENE: MUTYH

ASSOCIATED CANCERS: polyposis and colorectal cancer; possibly breast cancer, upper GI cancer, and endometrial cancer

MAP is caused when *both* copies of the MUTYH gene are broken (mutated). When *only one* copy is broken, a person is said to be a "carrier" of a MUTYH gene change. Information regarding cancer risks in MUTYH carriers is currently limited and conflicting. Recent studies have suggested that it may cause up to a twofold increased risk in colorectal cancer. Female carriers, particularly of North African Jewish ancestry, may have up to a 1.5-fold increased risk in breast cancer. Carriers of a MUTYH gene mutation are also at risk of passing that mutation on to their children. Since MAP is inherited in an autosomal recessive fashion (both copies of the gene need to be broken and inherited from carrier parents), it is possible to have MAP even if you have no family history of polyposis or cancer.

Patterns that suggest MAP include:

- Early-onset colorectal cancer at or under age forty
- Polyposis, when FAP is excluded
- Personal and family history of colorectal cancer and/or polyposis

Peutz-Jeghers Syndrome

ASSOCIATED GENE: STK11

ASSOCIATED CANCERS: breast cancer, colon cancer, gastric cancer, small bowel cancer, pancreatic cancer, ovarian cancer, cervical cancer, endometrial cancer, lung cancer, and tumors of the testes

People with Peutz-Jeghers syndrome will develop Peutz-Jeghers–type polyps (i.e., pathologists will examine and report polyps as being of the Peutz-Jeghers type). People often will also demonstrate unique staining and/or "freckling" of the lips, mouth, and gums as well as staining/freckling of the soles of the feet and palms of the hands.

Patterns that suggest Peutz-Jeghers syndrome include:

- Your doctor tells you that you have Peutz-Jeghers–type polyps
- Staining or freckling of the mouth, lips, nose, eyes, gums, genitalia, hands, or feet
- A personal or family history of cancers and clinical features associated with Peutz-Jeghers syndrome

Juvenile Polyposis Syndrome

ASSOCIATED GENES: BMPR1A and SMAD4

ASSOCIATED CANCERS: polyposis and colon cancer, stomach cancer, small bowel cancer, pancreatic cancer

People with SMAD4 mutations may also develop a separate genetic condition, hereditary hemorrhagic telangiectasia (HHT), characterized by development of abnormal blood vessels (telangiectasias) of the skin and other organs, which may lead to bleeding.

Patterns that suggest juvenile polyposis syndrome include:

- Any individual with juvenile-type polyps (i.e., pathologists examine and report the tumor as being a juvenile-type polyp)
- Personal and/or family history of cancers associated with juvenile polyposis syndrome
- Personal and/or family history of polyps and/or history of internal bleeding or dramatic and frequent nosebleeds
- Hereditary hemorrhagic telangiectasia syndrome (HHT)

Hereditary Leiomyomatosis Renal Cell Carcinoma Syndrome (HLRCC)

ASSOCIATED GENE: FH

ASSOCIATED CANCERS: renal cancer (most commonly type 2 papillary but a spectrum of renal tumors have been identified) and uterine leiomyosarcoma; possibly breast cancer, bladder cancer, Leydig cell tumors of the testis, and gastrointestinal stromal tumors (GISTs)

People with HLRCC also develop a benign type of tumor—called a leiomyoma—on the skin and in the uterus. Skin leiomyomas can be flesh-colored, red, or brown and may be sensitive to cold or touch. Uterine leiomyomas are also known as uterine fibroid tumors.

There are currently no established testing criteria for HLRCC, but you should consider testing in the following circumstances:

- Multiple leiomyomas (further evaluation should be considered even in the case of a single biopsy-confirmed leiomyoma of the skin)
- A personal and/or family history of leiomyomas *and* a personal and/or family history of renal carcinoma
- Early-onset type 2 papillary renal cell carcinoma

Birt-Hogg-Dubé Syndrome

ASSOCIATED GENE: FLCN

ASSOCIATED CANCERS: renal cancer (particularly oncocytoma and chromophobe pathology) and melanoma

People with Birt-Hogg-Dubé syndrome also are at risk for lung cysts and spontaneous lung collapse (known as pneumothorax), as well as skin findings such as fibrofolliculoma (a rash across the nose) and other unique skin lesions.

There are currently no established testing criteria for Birt-Hogg-Dubé syndrome, but you should consider testing in the following circumstances:

- Fibrofolliculoma (a bumpy rash on the nose)
- Skin findings such as fibrofolliculomas or other skin findings common in Birt-Hogg-Dubé syndrome (trichodiscomas and acrochordons), particularly if they have five or more facial/truncal lesions with at least one being confirmed as a fibrofolliculoma
- Oncocytoma or chromophobe-type renal cell carcinoma
- Renal cell carcinoma and/or skin findings associated with BHDS
- Multiple lung cysts
- Personal or family history of spontaneous lung collapse

c-MET

ASSOCIATED GENE: c-MET

ASSOCIATED CANCER RISKS: type 1 papillary renal cell carcinoma

There are currently no established testing criteria for c-MET, but you should consider testing under the following circumstances:

- Early-onset type 1 papillary renal cell carcinoma with or without a family history of renal cell carcinoma
- Individuals with a personal and family history of papillary renal cell carcinoma

Von Hippel–Lindau Syndrome (VHL)

ASSOCIATED GENE: VHL

ASSOCIATED CANCERS: hemangioblastomas of the retina and central nervous system, clear cell renal cell carcinoma, pheochromocytoma, pancreatic neuroendocrine tumors, and endolymphatic sac tumors

People with VHL may also develop cysts of the pancreas and kidneys.

Patterns that suggest VHL include:

- Personal or family history of hemangioblastoma, multiple renal cysts, renal cell carcinoma, pheochromocytoma, or endolymphatic sac tumor
- Clear cell renal cell carcinoma diagnosed below age fifty

HEREDITARY SKIN CANCER/MELANOMA PREDISPOSITION SYNDROMES

MITF

ASSOCIATED GENE: MITF

ASSOCIATED CANCERS: melanoma and renal cell carcinoma

There are currently no established testing criteria for MITF, but anyone who has had early-onset melanoma or early-onset renal cell carcinoma should consider a genetic risk assessment for MITF, particularly if there is a personal and/or family history of these cancers.

Familial Atypical Multiple Mole Melanoma Syndrome (FAMMM) and CDK4

ASSOCIATED GENES: CDKN2A and CDK4

ASSOCIATED CANCERS: melanoma and atypical moles; for CDKN2A mutations or FAMMM, breast and pancreatic cancers are possibly associated

There are currently no established testing criteria for CDKN2A or CDK4, but consider having a genetic risk assessment for these syndromes if you meet any of the following criteria:

- Early-onset melanoma in the absence of other risk factors (e.g., tanning, history of blistering sunburns)

- Three or more family members with melanoma, particularly early-onset
- Personal and/or family history of many atypical moles and/or melanoma
- Personal and/or family history of melanoma, breast cancer, and/or pancreatic cancer, particularly if early-onset

Gorlin Syndrome

ASSOCIATED GENE: PTCH1

ASSOCIATED CANCERS: basal cell carcinomas (particularly in sun- or radiation-exposed areas of the skin), cardiac and ovarian fibromas, and medulloblastoma

People with Gorlin syndrome may have additional clinical findings, including larger head size, skeletal abnormalities, and jaw cysts.

Patterns that suggest Gorlin syndrome include:

- Multiple or early-onset basal cell carcinomas
- Personal or family history of the clinical features characteristic of Gorlin syndrome, particularly if multiple features are present and/or occur at early ages

HEREDITARY ENDOCRINE TUMOR PREDISPOSITION SYNDROMES

Hereditary Pheochromocytoma Paraganglioma Syndrome (PGL-PCC)

ASSOCIATED GENES: SDHB, SDHD, SDHC, SDHA, SDHAF2, TMEM127, and MAX

ASSOCIATED CANCERS: pheochromocytoma, paraganglioma, renal cell carcinoma, and gastrointestinal stromal tumors (GISTs)

There are currently no established testing criteria for Hereditary PGL-PCC, but some studies suggest that up to 32 percent of apparently sporadic pheochromocytomas or paragangliomas may be due to an underlying hereditary predisposition. Consider genetic risk assessment and testing in all cases of paraganglioma or pheochromocytoma, particularly if any of the following are present:

- Multiple or bilateral tumors
- Multifocal tumors
- Recurrent tumors
- Early-onset tumors

Multiple Endocrine Neoplasia Type 1 (MEN1)

ASSOCIATED GENE: MEN1

ASSOCIATED CANCERS: parathyroid tumors, pancreatic tumors, pituitary tumors, carcinoid tumors (particularly thymus and the bronchi of the lung), and adrenocortical tumors

Non-endocrine tumors, including facial angiofibromas, collagenomas, lipomas, meningiomas, ependymomas, and leiomyomas may also be seen.

Patterns that suggest MEN1 include:

- Two or more tumors associated with cancers that can be caused by MEN1 syndrome
- One or more tumors associated with MEN1 *plus* a family history of tumors associated with MEN1, particularly if tumors are early-onset

Multiple Endocrine Neoplasia Type 2 (MEN2)

ASSOCIATED GENE: RET

ASSOCIATED CANCERS: medullary thyroid cancer and pheochromocytoma

Patterns that suggest MEN2 include:

- Medullary thyroid carcinoma at any age, regardless of family history

- Personal or family history of two or more clinical features associated with MEN2, including medullary thyroid cancer, pheochromocytoma, mucosal neuromas of the lips and/or tongue, ganglioneuromatosis of the GI tract, and/or primary hyperparathyroidism

PEDIATRIC CANCER PREDISPOSITION SYNDROMES

DICER1

ASSOCIATED GENE: DICER1

ASSOCIATED CANCERS: pleuropulmonary blastoma, ovarian sex cord-stromal tumors (Sertoli-Leydig cell tumor, juvenile granulosa cell tumors, gynandroblastoma), cystic nephroma, thyroid gland neoplasias, ciliary body medulloepitheliomas, botryoid-type embryonal rhabdomyosarcoma, nasal chondromesenchymal hamartomas, renal sarcoma, pituitary blastoma, pineoblastoma; rarely Wilms' tumor and neuroblastoma

There are currently no established testing criteria for DICER1, but testing should be considered for anyone with the following:

- Personal and/or family history of two or more of the cancers associated with DICER1 mutations
- Suspicious clinical features even in the absence of family history

Hereditary Retinoblastoma

ASSOCIATED GENE: RB1

ASSOCIATED CANCERS: retinoblastoma and pineoblastoma

Adult survivors of hereditary retinoblastoma are at increased risk for several malignancies, including melanoma, osteosarcoma, and soft-tissue sarcoma (primarily leiomyosarcoma and rhabdomyosarcoma). People with RB1 who are treated with radiation are at a particularly increased risk for second malignancies.

Patterns that suggest hereditary retinoblastoma:

- Retinoblastoma
- Bilateral retinoblastoma
- Family history of retinoblastoma

Fanconi Anemia

ASSOCIATED GENES: FANCA, FANCB, FANCC, BRCA2, FANCD2, FANCE, FANCF, FANCG, FANCI, BRIP1, FANCL, FANCM, PALB2, RAD51C, and SLX4

ASSOCIATED CANCERS: hematologic malignancies (particularly acute myeloid leukemia), cervical cancer, liver tumors, and squamous cell carcinomas of the head and neck, esophagus, and vulva

Many additional clinical features can be seen in people with Fanconi anemia syndrome, including short stature; birth defects; malformation of the thumbs or forearms, skeletal system, eyes, kidneys, urinary tract, ears, heart, GI system, and central nervous system; hypogonadism; and developmental delay. Many people with Fanconi anemia will develop progressive bone marrow failure. Some people with Fanconi anemia and no outward clinical features may not be diagnosed until they develop hematological problems or squamous cell cancers as adults.

Patterns that suggest Fanconi anemia include:

- Clinical features suggestive of the syndrome
- Thrombocytopenia, leukopenia, or progressive bone marrow failure, regardless of family history
- Early-onset squamous cell carcinoma

Note: Adults with undiagnosed Fanconi anemia may also present with exquisite sensitivity to chemotherapy during cancer treatments

Neurofibromatosis Type 1 (NF1)

ASSOCIATED GENE: NF1

ASSOCIATED CANCERS: neurofibromas, plexiform neurofibromas, and optic gliomas; possibly breast cancer

Patterns that suggest NF1 include:

* Two or more neurofibromas or one or more plexiform neurofibromas
* Six or more café-au-lait birthmarks
* Axillary freckling (freckles in the groin or armpits)
* Optic gliomas
* Two or more Lisch nodules (a benign freckle in the eye)
* Bone lesions such as sphenoid dysplasia or thinning of long bone cortex
* Family history of NF1

Tuberous Sclerosis Complex (TSC)

ASSOCIATED GENES: TSC1 and TSC2

ASSOCIATED CANCERS: brain, spine, kidney, or cardiac tumors

People with TSC can have many other clinical features, including characteristic skin findings, renal cysts, and bone cysts.

Patterns that suggest TSC:

* Any individuals with any major feature of TSC or two or more minor features of TSC

Wilms' Tumor 1 (WT1) Syndromes: WAGR, Denys-Drash, Frasier

ASSOCIATED GENE: WT1

ASSOCIATED CANCERS: Wilms' tumor

Patterns that suggest WT1 include:

* Unusually early-onset, bilateral, or multicentric Wilms' tumors
* Family history of Wilms' tumor

- People with WT1 associated Wilms' tumors may also have one of the following syndromes.
  - WAGR syndrome: Wilms' tumor, aniridia, genital anomalies, retardation
  - Denys-Drash syndrome: undermasculinized external genitalia, early-onset renal failure
  - Frasier syndrome: undermasculinized external genitalia, focal segmental glomerulosclerosis, gonadoblastoma

Beckwith-Wiedemann Syndrome

ASSOCIATED GENES: Several unique genetic mechanisms are known to be responsible for Beckwith-Wiedemann syndrome, including methylation of the maternal IC1 or IC2, maternal CDKN1C mutations, paternal uniparental disomy (UPD) of 11p15.5, and other genomic alterations at 11p15.5.

ASSOCIATED CANCERS: Wilms' tumor, hepatoblastoma, neuroblastoma, and rhabdomyosarcoma

People with Beckwith-Wiedemann syndrome usually have several other clinical features, including an enlarged mouth and tongue, enlarged visceral organs, ophalocele, hypoglycemia, ear creases/pits, and kidney abnormalities.

Anyone with clinical features suggestive of Beckwith-Wiedemann syndrome should be evaluated further. This syndrome is usually diagnosed in infancy or early childhood.

Carney Complex

ASSOCIATED GENE: PRKAR1A

ASSOCIATED CANCERS: myxomas, large-cell calcifying Sertoli cell tumors, endocrine tumors, schwannomas, growth-hormone-producing adenomas

People with Carney complex may have several other clinical features, including skin pigmentary abnormalities, adrenocortical disease, Cushing's syndrome, and thyroid nodules.

Patterns that suggest Carney complex include:

- Spotty skin pigmentation with specific distribution (lips, conjunctiva and inner or outer canthi, vaginal and penile mucosal)
- Unique tumors of the skin, mouth, heart, breast, adrenal glands, pituitary gland, testes, thyroid, and bone
- Blue nevus (unique blue birthmarks)
- Intense freckling (without darkly pigmented spots or typical distribution)
- Café-au-lait spots or other birthmarks
- Cardiomyopathy
- Pilonidal sinus
- History of Cushing's syndrome, acromegaly, or sudden death in extended family
- Multiple skin tags or other skin lesions; lipomas
- Colonic polyps (usually in association with acromegaly)
- Hyperprolactinemia (usually mild and almost always combined with clinical or subclinical acromegaly)
- Single, benign thyroid nodule in a child younger than age eighteen years; multiple thyroid nodules in an individual older than age eighteen years (detected on ultrasound examination)
- Family history of carcinoma, in particular of the thyroid, colon, pancreas, and ovary; other multiple benign or malignant tumors

Rhabdoid Tumor Predisposition

ASSOCIATED GENES: INI1 and SMARCB1

ASSOCIATED CANCERS: rhabdoid tumors (particularly atypical teratoid/rhabdoid tumor of the central nervous system and malignant renal rhabdoid tumors), schwannomatosis

Patterns that suggest rhabdoid tumor predisposition include:

- Malignant rhabdoid tumor
- Personal and/or family history of schwannomatosis

Xeroderma Pigmentosum

ASSOCIATED GENES: XPA, ERCC1, ERCC3, XPC, ERCC2, DDB2, ERCC4, ERCC5, and POLH

ASSOCIATED CANCERS: skin cancer (basal cell carcinoma, squamous cell carcinoma, and melanoma)

Patterns that suggest xeroderma pigmentosum include:

- Extreme sun sensitivity (blistering and redness with minimal sun exposure)
- Marked freckle-like pigmentation before the age of two
- Eye problems (sensitivity to light, keratitis, atrophy of the eyelids)
- Progressive neurological problems
- Early-onset or multiple skin cancers

Shwachman-Diamond Syndrome

ASSOCIATED GENE: SBDS

ASSOCIATED CANCERS: myelodysplastic syndrome and acute myelogenous leukemia (AML)

Patterns that suggest Shwachman-Diamond syndrome include:

- Hematological abnormalities (most commonly MDS, AML, neutropenia, and cytopenia), particularly if there is also a personal history of:
  - Pancreatic dysfunction and/or malabsorption, malnutrition, and growth failure
  - Bone abnormalities
  - Short stature
  - Recurrent infections
- Family history of pancreatic problems, growth problems, or blood abnormalities

Diamond-Blackfan Anemia

ASSOCIATED GENES: Several genes are mutated in DBA and most encode for ribosomal proteins. RPS19 is the most commonly mutated gene (found in 25 percent of DBA patients).

ASSOCIATED CANCERS: myelodysplastic syndrome, acute myelogenous leukemia (AML), and solid tumors, including osteogenic sarcoma

Patterns that suggest Diamond-Blackfan anemia include:

* Profound anemia with normal white blood cells and platelets
* Birth defects (craniofacial, upper-limb, heart, and genitourinary)
* Growth retardation
* Fetal anemia with nonimmune hydrops fetalis
* Family history of birth defects or hematological abnormalities

Dyskeratosis Congenita

ASSOCIATED GENES: CTC1, DKC1, TERC, TERT, TINF2, NHP2, NOP10, and WRAP53

ASSOCIATED CANCERS: myelodysplastic syndrome, acute myelogenous leukemia (AML), and solid tumors, including squamous cell carcinomas of the head and neck and anogenital cancers

Patterns that suggest dyskeratosis congenita include:

* Any of the above cancers
* Absent or underformed nails
* Lacy reticular pigmentation of the upper chest and/or neck
* Oral leukoplakia (characteristic white patches in the mouth)
* Progressive bone marrow failure
* Pulmonary fibrosis
* Other abnormal pigmentation findings
* Eye abnormalities
* Dental abnormalities
* Developmental delay

APPENDIX 2

Risk Management for
Inherited Cancer Syndromes

RISK MANAGEMENT FOR INHERITED CANCER SYNDROMES

Inherited Cancer Syndrome	Lifetime Cancer Risks	Current Management Guidelines, Women	Current Management Guidelines, Men
Hereditary Breast and Ovarian Cancer Syndrome (BRCA1, BRCA2)	Female breast cancer (45–87%) Male breast cancer (BRCA1, 1–1.2%; BRCA2, 6–6.8%) Ovarian cancer (BRCA1, 40%; BRCA2, 18%) Prostate cancer (20–30%) Pancreas cancer (BRCA1, 1–4%; BRCA2, 6%) Melanoma: increased Colon and gastric cancer: increased	• Breast "self-awareness" beginning by age 18 (defined by the National Comprehensive Cancer Network as being familiar with your breasts and promptly reporting anything unusual to your physicians; NCCN also states that breast self-exams may help "facilitate" breast self-awareness) • Clinical breast exam every 6–12 months beginning by age 25 or 5–10 years younger than the age of youngest breast cancer diagnosis in the family • Annual breast MRI screening by age 25–29 or individualized based on the youngest age of diagnosis in the family (breast mammogram can be considered if MRI is unavailable) • Annual mammogram alternating with breast MRI every 6 months beginning by age >30–75. After age 75, breast screening should be considered on an individual basis.	• Breast self-exam education and training beginning by age 35 • Clinical breast exam every 6–12 months beginning by age 35 • Baseline mammogram at age 40 can be considered • Annual mammogram can be considered in men with gynecomastia (extra breast tissue) or breast density • Begin annual prostate cancer screening by age 40 or 10 years younger than the age of the youngest diagnosis in the family • Currently no management guidelines for colon, gastric, or pancreatic cancer

Hereditary Breast and Ovarian Cancer Syndrome (BRCA1, BRCA2) *(continued)*	• Consider prophylactic mastectomy • Consider chemoprevention such as tamoxifen and oral birth control pills • Consider PARP inhibitors for ovarian cancer patients • Risk-reducing removal of the ovaries (bilateral salpingo-oophorectomy) can be recommended for women who have completed childbearing and have reached at least age 35 • Ovarian screening consisting of transvaginal ultrasound and CA-125 every 6 months may be considered • Consider annual dermatological and ophthalmological exam for melanoma • Currently no surveillance or management guidelines for colon, gastric, or pancreatic cancers

Inherited Cancer Syndrome	Lifetime Cancer Risks	Current Management Guidelines, Women	Current Management Guidelines, Men

Li-Fraumeni Syndrome (TP53)	**Lifetime risk of any cancer:**
	
	50% by age 30
	90% by age 60
	
	Relative risk by tumor type:
	
	Osteosarcoma (107)
	Sarcoma (61)
	Brain (35)
	Pancreas (7.3)
	Breast (6.4)
	Colon (2.8)
	Liver (1.8)
		• Annual physical examination by a doctor including careful neurological and dermatological examinations
		• High-risk breast cancer surveillance
		  • Clinical breast exam every 6–12 months starting at age 20–25 or 10 years younger than the earliest known breast cancer in the family
		  • Annual mammogram and breast MRI screening starting at age 20–25 or individualized based on the earliest age of onset in the family
		  • Women under age 30 may consider breast MRI only with addition of breast mammogram after age 30 (see breast cancer section below for details)
		  • Consideration of prophylactic risk-reducing mastectomy
		• High-risk colorectal cancer surveillance
		  • Colonoscopy every 2–5 years starting no later than age 25
			Screening recommendations for men are the same as those for women, with exception of breast management

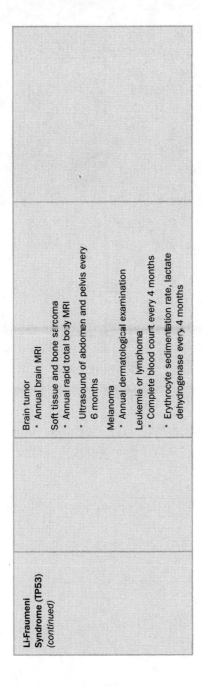

| Li-Fraumeni Syndrome (TP53) (continued) | | Brain tumor
• Annual brain MRI

Soft tissue and bone sarcoma
• Annual rapid total body MRI
• Ultrasound of abdomen and pelvis every 6 months

Melanoma
• Annual dermatological examination

Leukemia or lymphoma
• Complete blood count every 4 months
• Erythrocyte sedimentation rate, lactate dehydrogenase every 4 months | |

Inherited Cancer Syndrome	Lifetime Cancer Risks	Current Management Guidelines, Women	Current Management Guidelines, Men
Li-Fraumeni Syndrome (TP53) *(continued)*		**CHILDREN** Adrenocortical carcinoma • Ultrasound of abdomen and pelvis every 3–4 months • Complete urinalysis every 3–4 months • Blood tests every 4 months: beta-human chorionic gonadotropin, alpha-fetoprotein, 17-OH-progesterone, testosterone, dehydroepiandrosterone sulfate, androstenedione Brain tumor • Annual brain MRI Soft tissue and bone sarcoma • Annual rapid total body MRI Leukemia or lymphoma • Blood test every 4 months: complete blood count, erythrocyte sedimentation rate, lactate dehydrogenase	

Inherited Cancer Syndrome	Lifetime Cancer Risks	Current Management Guidelines, Women	Current Management Guidelines, Men
ATM (heterozygous) mutation)* **Note:** People with homozygous (both ATM genes abnormal) ATM gene mutations have a syndrome known as ataxia-telangiectasia	Breast (28–50%) Pancreas: increased, exact risks unknown Possible increased risks: prostate, melanoma, endometrial, head and neck, hematological malignancies	• Annual breast MRI screening by age 25–29 or individualized based on the youngest age of diagnosis in the family (mammogram can be considered if MRI is unavailable) • Annual mammogram alternating with breast MRI every 6 months beginning by age >30–75. After age 75, screening is individualized.	Currently no established screening or management guidelines for men with heterozygous ATM gene mutations
BARD1, BRIP1, MRE11A, RAD50, RAD51C, RAD51D†	Breast (up to ~36%) Ovarian cancer: possibly increased (~9% in RAD51C and ~10% in RAD51D, exact lifetime risks unknown with others)	• Consider discussing high risk breast and ovarian management with your doctor	Currently no established screening and management guidelines for men

Inherited Cancer Syndrome	Lifetime Cancer Risks	Current Management Guidelines, Women	Current Management Guidelines, Men
CHEK2 (heterozygous mutations)*	Breast cancer (20–25%) Colon cancer: increased Prostate cancer (27%) Possible increased risks: ovarian cancer, thyroid cancer, renal cancer	• Annual breast MRI screening by age 25–29 or individualized based on the youngest age of diagnosis in the family (breast mammogram can be considered if MRI is unavailable) • Annual mammogram alternating with breast MRI every 6 months beginning by age >30–75. After age 75, breast screening should be considered on an individual basis	Consider beginning prostate cancer surveillance with DRE and PSA beginning by age 40 or 10 years younger than the age of the youngest diagnosis in the family, whichever is earlier
NBN (heterozygous mutations)†	Breast cancer (up to ~36%) Possibly ovarian cancer	• Currently no established screening and management guidelines for women with heterozygous NBN gene mutations	Currently no established screening and management guidelines for men with heterozygous NBN gene mutations

Inherited Cancer Syndrome	Lifetime Cancer Risks	Current Management Guidelines, Women	Current Management Guidelines, Men
PALB2 (heterozygous mutations)*	Breast cancer (24–48%) Pancreatic cancer: increased Possibly ovarian cancer	• Annual breast MRI screening by age 25–29 or individualized based on the youngest age of diagnosis in the family (breast mammogram can be considered if MRI is unavailable) • Annual mammogram alternating with breast MRI every 6 months beginning by age >30–75. After age 75, breast screening should be considered on an individual basis • Currently no surveillance or management guidelines for pancreatic cancer	Currently no established screening and management guidelines for men with heterozygous PALB2 gene mutations

Inherited Cancer Syndrome	Lifetime Cancer Risks	Current Management Guidelines, Women	Current Management Guidelines, Men
Cowden Syndrome (PTEN)	Breast cancer (50–85%) Thyroid cancer (10–35%) Endometrial cancer (10–28%) Renal cancer (up to 35%) Colon cancer: increased	• Breast awareness starting at age 18 • Clinical breast exams every 6–12 months starting at age 25 or 5–10 years younger than the age of the youngest breast cancer diagnosis in the family • Annual mammogram and breast MRI starting at age 30–35 or 5–10 years younger than the age of the youngest breast cancer diagnosis in the family. After age 75, breast screening should be considered on an individual basis • Encourage patient education of and prompt response to possible symptoms of endometrial cancer • Consider annual random endometrial biopsy and/or ultrasound beginning by age 30–35 • Discuss option of risk-reducing mastectomy and hysterectomy • Annual comprehensive physical exam starting at age 18 or 5 years before the youngest age of diagnosis of a Cowden syndrome-related cancer in the family with particular attention to a thyroid exam	• Annual comprehensive physical exam starting at age 18 or 5 years before the youngest age of diagnosis of a Cowden syndrome-related cancer in the family with particular attention to a thyroid exam • Annual thyroid ultrasound starting at the time of diagnosis • Colonoscopy starting at age 35 or unless symptomatic or with a relative diagnosed under the age of 40 • Colonoscopy should be done every 5 years or more frequently if patient is symptomatic or polyps are found • Consider dermatological management • Consider psychomotor assessment in children at diagnosis and brain MRI if there are symptoms

Cowden Syndrome (PTEN) *(continued)*		• Annual thyroid ultrasound starting at the time of diagnosis • Colonoscopy starting at age 35 or unless symptomatic or with a relative diagnosed under the age of 40; colonoscopy should be done every 5 years or more frequently if patient is symptomatic or polyps are found • Consider dermatological management • Consider psychomotor assessment in children at diagnosis and brain MRI if there are symptoms

Inherited Cancer Syndrome	Lifetime Cancer Risks	Current Management Guidelines, Women	Current Management Guidelines, Men
Familial Adenomatous Polyposis (APC)	Colon cancer (100% by age 45 without intervention)	• Screening with colonoscopy annually beginning at ages 10–15	See female guidelines
	Small bowel cancer (4–12%)	• Colectomy, the timing of which will depend on onset and number of polyposis	
	Gastric cancer (1%)	• Continued surveillance of rectum and pouch, frequency depending on surgery performed and polyp burden	
	Pancreas cancer (2%)		
	Thyroid cancer (1–12%)	• Based upper endoscopy with side-viewing scope	
	Hepatoblastoma (1–1.6% to age 5)	• Annual thyroid exam beginning in late teenage years	
	CNS cancer (~1%)	• Annual abdominal palpation and physical exam for desmoids; if strong family history of desmoids, abdominal MRI or CT scan can be considered	
	Desmoid tumors (13%)		
	Bile duct/adrenal gland cancer: increased	• Patients should inform physicians of any unusual lumps, bumps, or pain	
		• Liver palpation, abdominal ultrasound, and AFP levels every 3–6 months in children age ≤5	
		• Currently no recommended guidelines for pancreatic or CNS screening	

Inherited Cancer Syndrome	Lifetime Cancer Risks	Current Management Guidelines, Women	Current Management Guidelines, Men
Hereditary Diffuse Gastric Cancer (CDH1)	Gastric cancer (67–83%) Lobular breast cancer (39–60%) Possibly colon cancer	• Baseline endoscopy at time of diagnosis • Consider prophylactic gastrectomy • For individuals who decline gastrectomy, annual endoscopy with special precautions for diffuse-type gastric cancer • Breast awareness starting at age 18 • Clinical breast exams every 6–12 months starting at age 25 or 5–10 years younger than the age of the youngest breast cancer diagnosis in the family • Annual mammogram and breast MRI starting at age 30–35 or 5–10 years younger than the age of the youngest breast cancer diagnosis in the family. After age 75 breast screening should be considered on an individual basis. • Consider screening colonoscopy by age 40 or 10 years younger than the youngest age of colon cancer diagnosis in the family. Colonoscopy should be repeated every 3–5 years.	See female guidelines

Inherited Cancer Syndrome	Lifetime Cancer Risks	Current Management Guidelines, Women	Current Management Guidelines, Men
Lynch Syndrome (MLH1, MSH2, MSH6, PMS2, EPCAM)	Female colon cancer (30–52%) Male colon cancer (50–74%) Endometrial cancer (28–71%) Ovarian cancer (9–12%) Gastric cancer (5–8%) CNS tumors (3%) Small bowel cancer (1–4%) Pancreatic cancer (6%) Bladder/ureter cancer (1–4%) Hepatobiliary cancer (1–4%) Renal cancer: increased Breast cancer: possibly increased	For MLH1, MSH2, and EPCAM mutation carriers: • Colonoscopy at age 20–25 or 2–5 years younger than the age of the youngest colon cancer diagnosis in the family; repeat every 1–2 years • Consider risk-reducing hysterectomy and removal of the ovaries (bilateral salpingo-oophorectomy) after childbearing • Currently no sufficient evidence for uterine or ovarian cancer screening, but may be considered at a clinician's discretion • Currently no clear evidence to support screening for gastric, duodenal, and small bowel cancers. Selected individuals or families or those of Asian descent may consider esophagogastroduodenoscopy with extended duodenoscopy every 3–5 years beginning at age 30–35. • Consider annual urinalysis beginning at age 25–30 • Annual physical/neurological exam beginning by age 25–30 • Currently no established screening guidelines for pancreatic cancer or breast cancer	See female guidelines

Lynch Syndrome (MLH1, MSH2, MSH6, PMS2, EPCAM) *(continued)*		For MSH6 and PMS2 mutation carriers • Colonoscopy at age 25–30 or 2–5 years younger than the age of the youngest colon cancer diagnosis in the family if it is diagnosed before age 30; repeat every 1–2 years • Consider risk-reducing hysterectomy and removal of the ovaries (bilateral salpingo-oophorectomy) after childbearing • Currently no sufficient evidence for uterine or ovarian cancer screening, but may be considered at a clinician's discretion • Risk of other Lynch syndrome–related cancers is reportedly low; however, due to limited data, no screening recommendations exist at this time

Inherited Cancer Syndrome	Lifetime Cancer Risks	Current Management Guidelines, Women	Current Management Guidelines, Men
Peutz-Jeghers Syndrome (STK11)	Breast cancer (45–50%) Colon cancer (39%) Gastric cancer (29%) Small intestine cancer (13%) Pancreas cancer (11–36%) Ovarian cancer (18–21%) Cervical cancer (10%) Uterine cancer (9%) Lung cancer (15–17%) Testicular cancer: increased	• Clinical breast exam every 6 months beginning by age 25 • Annual mammogram and breast MRI beginning by age 25 • Colonoscopy every 2–3 years beginning in late teens • Upper endoscopy every 2–3 years beginning in late teens • Small bowel screening with CT scan or MRI enterography baseline at 8–10 years with follow-up interval based on age. Then every 2–3 years beginning by age 18. • Magnetic resonance cholangiopancreatography or endoscopic ultrasound every 1–2 years beginning by age 30–35 • Annual pelvic exam and Pap smear beginning by age 18–20 • Consider transvaginal ultrasound • Currently no screening recommendations for lung cancer; consider smoking cessation	• See female guidelines • Annual testicular exam and observation for feminizing changes beginning by age 10

Inherited Cancer Syndrome	Lifetime Cancer Risks	Current Management Guidelines, Women	Current Management Guidelines, Men
Juvenile Polyposis Syndrome (BMPR1A, SMAD4)	Colon cancer (40–50%) Gastric cancer (21% if significant polyposis) Small bowel cancer: increased Pancreas cancer: increased	• Colonoscopy beginning by age 15; repeat annually if polyps and every 2–3 years if no polyps • Upper endoscopy beginning by age 15; repeat annually if polyps and every 2–3 years if no polyps • In individuals with SMAD4 mutations, screen for vascular lesions associated with hereditary hemorrhagic telangiectasia beginning in the first 6 months of life • Currently no screening and management guidelines for small bowel or pancreatic cancer	See female guidelines

Inherited Cancer Syndrome	Lifetime Cancer Risks	Current Management Guidelines, Women	Current Management Guidelines, Men
Hereditary Leiomyomatosis Renal Cell Carcinoma Syndrome (FH)*	Renal cancer (up to 20%) Leiomyosarcoma: increased Possibly breast cancer, bladder cancer, Leydig-cell tumors of the testis, and gastrointestinal stromal tumors	• Full skin examination is recommended annually to every 2 years to assess the extent of disease and to evaluate for changes suggestive of leiomyosarcoma • Annual gynecologic consultation is recommended to assess severity of uterine fibroids and to evaluate for changes suggestive of leiomyosarcoma • Yearly examination with abdominal MRI or CT scan with and without contrast are recommended for individuals with normal initial baseline or follow-up abdominal MRI or CT scan. MRI may be preferred because of the potential added lifetime radiation exposure associated with CT scan • Any suspicious renal lesion (indeterminate lesion, questionable or complex cysts) at a previous examination should be followed with a CT scan with and without contrast. The use of renal ultrasound examination is helpful in the characterization of cystic lesions. PET-CT scan may be added to identify metabolically active lesions suggesting possible malignant growth. Caution: Ultrasound examination alone is never sufficient. • Renal tumors should be evaluated by a urologic oncology surgeon familiar with the renal cancer of HLRCC	See female guidelines

Inherited Cancer Syndrome	Lifetime Cancer Risks	Current Management Guidelines, Women	Current Management Guidelines, Men
Birt-Hogg-Dubé Syndrome (FLCN)*	Renal cancer (up to 34%) Melanoma: increased	• Consider annual pelvic MRI for renal cancer screening beginning by age 18 • Renal tumors less than 3 centimeters in diameter are monitored by periodic imaging. When the largest renal tumor reaches 3 centimeters in maximal diameter, evaluation by a urologic surgeon is appropriate with consideration of nephron-sparing surgery.	See female guidelines
c-MET (heterozygous mutations)†	Renal cancer: increased	Currently no consensus guidelines for screening and management for c-MET mutations Consider discussing screening options for kidney cancer with your doctor	See female guidelines

Inherited Cancer Syndrome	Lifetime Cancer Risks	Current Management Guidelines, Women	Current Management Guidelines, Men
Von Hippel–Lindau Syndrome (VHL)	Renal cancer (25–60%) CNS hemangioblastoma (13–72%) Retinal hemangioblastoma (25–60%) Endolymphatic sac tumors (15%) Pheochromocytoma (10–20%) Pancreatic cysts/lesions (35–60%) Cystadenomas of the epididymis (25–60%) Cystadenomas of the broad ligament (10%)	• Annual evaluation starting at age 1 for neurological symptoms, vision problems, or hearing disturbances • Annual exam starting at age 1 for signs of nystagmus, strabismus (gaze disturbances), or white pupils • Annual blood pressure monitoring starting at age 1 • Annual ophthalmology exam with indirect ophthalmoscope starting at age 1 • Annual blood or urinary fractionated metanephrines starting at age 5 • Audiology assessment every 2–3 years (annually if hearing loss, ear ringing, or vertigo) starting at age 5 • Annual abdominal ultrasound and every other year MRI scan of the abdomen beginning at age 16 • MRI of the brain and total spine every 2 years starting at age 16 with attention given to the inner ear/petrous temporal bone and posterior fossa	See female guidelines

Inherited Cancer Syndrome	Lifetime Cancer Risks	Current Management Guidelines, Women	Current Management Guidelines, Men
MITF (heterozygous mutations)[†]	Melanoma: increased Renal cell carcinoma: increased Individuals with the p.E318K mutation have ≥ fivefold increased risk for melanoma, RCC, or both	Currently no established screening and management guidelines for heterozygous MITF mutations Consider discussing screening options for kidney cancer and dermatological exam with your doctor	See female guidelines
Familial Atypical Multiple Mole Melanoma Syndrome (FAMMM)/CDKN2A (heterozygous mutations)[†]	Melanoma (28–67%) Pancreas (17–58%)	Currently no established screening and management guidelines for heterozygous P16 mutations Consider discussing dermatological examination with your doctor	See female guidelines
CDK4 (heterozygous mutations)[†]	Melanoma (74%)	Currently no established screening and management guidelines for heterozygous CDK4 mutations Consider discussing dermatological examination with your doctor	See female guidelines

Inherited Cancer Syndrome	Lifetime Cancer Risks	Current Management Guidelines, Women	Current Management Guidelines, Men
Gorlin Syndrome (PTCH1)*	Basal cell carcinoma: significantly increased Medulloblastoma (1–5%) Cardiac fibromas (~2%) Ovarian fibromas (~20%)	• Head circumference should be followed through childhood • Baseline physical exam for birth defects of clinical significance • X-rays to evaluate for rib and vertebral anomalies and calcification of the falx • Ophthalmological exam for evidence of cataracts and developmental defects • Echocardiogram in the first year of life to evaluate for cardiac fibromas • Orthopentogram every 12–18 months in individuals age >8 • Dermatology exam at least annually	See female guidelines

Inherited Cancer Syndrome	Lifetime Cancer Risks	Current Management Guidelines, Women	Current Management Guidelines, Men
Hereditary Pheochromocytoma Paraganglioma Syndrome (SDHB, SDHD, SDHC, SDHA, SDHAF2, TMEM127, MAX)	Paraganglioma (up to 100%) Pheochromocytoma (up to 100%) Gastrointestinal stromal tumor: increased, particularly in SDHA, SDHB, and SDHD Renal cell carcinoma: increased, particularly in SDHB	• Screening should begin at age 10 or at least 10 years younger than the earliest age at diagnosis in the family • 24-hour urine fractionated metanephrines and catecholamines and/or plasma fractionated metanephrines • Follow-up imaging by MRI, CT scan, 123I-MIBG, or FDG-PET if the metanephrine or catecholamine levels become elevated • MRI or CT scan of the skull base and neck every 2 years and MRI or CT scan and 123I-MIBG scintigraphy of the body every 4 years in individuals with SDHD or SDHC mutations • MRI or CT scan of the abdomen, thorax, and pelvis every 2 years and 123I-MIBG scintigraphy every 4 years in individuals with SDHB mutations with particular attention to the kidneys	See female guidelines

Inherited Cancer Syndrome	Lifetime Cancer Risks	Current Management Guidelines, Women	Current Management Guidelines, Men
Multiple Endocrine Neoplasia Type 1 (MEN1)	Parathyroid (~100% by age 50) Pituitary (~10–60%) Pancreatic/GEP tumors (30–80%) Carcinoid (10%) Adrenocortical (~20–40%) Meningioma (~8%) Ependymoma (1%)	• Annual serum concentration of prolactin, IGF-1, fasting glucose, and insulin beginning at age 5 • Annual fasting total serum calcium concentration, chromogranin-A, pancreatic polypeptide, glucagon, vasoactive intestinal peptide for other pancreatic neuroendocrine tumors beginning by age 8 • Annual fasting serum gastrin concentration by age 20 • Consider annual fasting serum concentration of intact (full-length) PTH • Head MRI every 3–5 years beginning by age 5 • Abdominal CT scan or MRI every 3–5 years beginning by age 20 • Consider annual chest CT scan • Consider annual somatostatin receptor scintigraphy octreotide scan	See female guidelines

Inherited Cancer Syndrome	Lifetime Cancer Risks	Current Management Guidelines, Women	Current Management Guidelines, Men
Multiple Endocrine Neoplasia Type 2 (RET)	Medullary thyroid cancer (95–100%) Pheochromocytoma (50%)	• Prophylactic thyroidectomy (removal of the thyroid) as directed by mutation level • Annual biochemical thyroid screening for individuals who have not undergone thyroidectomy • Annual serum calcitonin beginning at age 6 months for individuals with MEN2B and age 3–5 for individuals with MEN2A or FMTC • Annual measurement of serum calcitonin in all individuals after thyroidectomy • Annual biochemical screening for pheochromocytoma beginning by age 8 with follow-up with MRI or CT scan if biochemical screening is abnormal • Annual biochemical parathyroid screening for individuals who have not undergone parathyroidectomy	See female guidelines

Inherited Cancer Syndrome	Lifetime Cancer Risks	Current Management Guidelines, Women	Current Management Guidelines, Men
DICER1 (heterozygous mutations)*	**Lifetime risk of any cancer:** ~50% in females ~20% in males Pleuropulmonary blastoma, ovarian sex-cord stromal tumors, cystic nephroma, nodular hyperplasia of the thyroid, ciliary body medulloepithelioma, botryoid-type embryonal rhabdomyosarcoma, nasal chondromesenchymal hamartoma, pituitary blastoma, and pineoblastoma: increased. Exact lifetime risks unknown. Age of onset of tumors also may vary.	Consider annual physical examination and targeted review of systems with imaging study type and frequency based on tumor type, patient age, and suspicious clinical findings. • Consider baseline chest CT scan to evaluate for lung cysts—critical age group for PPB is below age 3 • Consider baseline kidney CT scan or ultrasound examination in individuals diagnosed with PPB • Consider annual abdominal exam and monitoring for pain or swelling, particularly in patients younger than 4 • Consider thyroid physical exam with thyroid sonogram every 3–5 years • Consider examination of all females at any age for signs and symptoms of precocious puberty or virilization and masses in the abdomen or pelvis • Consider abdominal and pelvic imaging • Consider laboratory testing for ovarian stromal tumors • Consider evaluation of young children for ciliary body medulloepithelioma with visual inspection of eye and orbit and measurement of visual acuity	See female guidelines

DICER1 (heterozygous mutations) (continued)		• Consider endoscopic evaluation of the bladder or direct visualization of cervix in individuals with hematuria or abnormal vaginal bleeding for potential botryoid ERMS • Consider nasal endoscopy if concerns for NCMH • Consider brain MRI for pituitary blastoma or pineoblastoma, especially if signs of cortical excess or increased intracranial pressure

Inherited Cancer Syndrome	Lifetime Cancer Risks	Current Management Guidelines, Women	Current Management Guidelines, Men
Hereditary Retinoblastoma (RB1)	Retinoblastoma: increased Pinealoblastoma: rare, but increased Second malignancies in adult individuals: increased, particularly melanoma and sarcoma and particularly in people who have undergone radiation treatment	• People with a known RB1 germline mutation should undergo eye exam under anesthesia every 3–4 weeks until age 6 months, then less frequently until age 3. They should undergo clinical eye exams every 3–6 months until age 7, then annually and eventually biannually for life. • People at risk for a potential RB1 mutation (e.g., children of people with a history of retinoblastoma) who have tested negative for RB1 gene mutations should consider examination by an ophthalmologist familiar with retinoblastoma shortly after birth and should have eye exams with attention for red reflex at routine pediatric visits • Currently no established surveillance and management guidelines for other cancers that may be seen in adults with hereditary retinoblastoma; consider annual dermatological evaluation and promptly report any lumps, bumps, or pain to physician for further evaluation	See female guidelines

Inherited Cancer Syndrome	Lifetime Cancer Risks	Current Management Guidelines — Women	Current Management Guidelines, Men
Fanconi Anemia	**Cumulative incidence by age 50:** Hematological malignancies (10–30%) Bone marrow failure (90%) Squamous cell tumors of the head and neck, skin, GI tract, and genital tract (25–30%)	• Monitor growth and pubertal development closely with referral to endocrinologist if indicated • Blood counts every 2–3 months or more frequently if needed • Bone marrow aspirate/biopsy at least annually • For people receiving androgen therapy: regular monitoring of liver chemistry profile and ultrasound exam of the liver every 6–12 months • Annual gynecologic exam and Pap smears beginning at menarche or age 16, whichever is earlier • Frequent dental and oropharyngeal exams including nasolaryngoscopy beginning by age 10 • Consider annual esophageal endoscopy	See female guidelines

Inherited Cancer Syndrome	Lifetime Cancer Risks	Current Management Guidelines, Women	Current Management Guidelines, Men
Neurofibromatosis type 1 (NF1)	Neurofibromas: significantly increased Breast cancer (up to ~60%)	• Annual physical exam • Annual ophthalmological exam in childhood, less frequently in older children and adults • Regular developmental assessment in childhood • Regular blood pressure monitoring • Currently no consensus screening guidelines for breast cancer in women with NF1	See female guidelines

* There is currently no comprehensive consensus on clinical surveillance and management for this syndrome. However, some surveillance and/or management guidelines have been developed by various clinical organizations for some clinical aspects of the syndrome. Those guidelines are listed here.

† There are currently no clinical surveillance or management guidelines for this syndrome. Surveillance and management should be determined by treating physicians based on personal and/or family history and clinical situation.

RESOURCES

CANCER AND GENETICS GENERAL INFORMATION

NOTE: This is only a sampling of many available Web resources.

American Cancer Society

The American Cancer Society website has many general resources related to cancer, updates on genetics, and patient support.

www.cancer.org

Cancer and Careers

This website addresses many issues related to dealing with cancer treatment in the workplace. It includes strategies for discussing your diagnosis with your employer, including navigating necessary time off and insurance, traveling, and advice about how to "keep up appearances" during cancer treatment.

www.cancerandcareers.org

Genetic Alliance

Genetic Alliance is a nonprofit that advocates for patients' rights in genetic health issues and provides information.

www.geneticalliance.org

Genetics Home Reference

This is a site that offers a patient-friendly explanation of genetic syndromes. It also provides additional websites and resources.

http://ghr.nlm.nih.gov

Cancer101

This is a patient advocacy organization that provides tools and resources for patients and caregivers to navigate the cancer journey to make informed medical decisions. The best part of this site is the C101 planner, which empowers patients with information, engages them to take control of their diagnosis, and helps them stay organized.

www.cancer101.org

Cancer Support Community

Completely free of charge and nonprofit, Cancer Support Community offers support groups, networking groups, lectures, workshops, and social events in a nonresidential, homelike setting. If you, a family member, or a friend has cancer, please explore this website to discover a program that will give you the social and emotional support that you need.

http://www.cancersupportcommunity.org

National Society of Genetic Counselors

This website introduces genetic counseling and offers much information, including how to find a genetic counselor near you.

http://www.nsgc.org

HEREDITARY BREAST AND OVARIAN
CANCER SYNDROME (HBOC)

These links are useful for patients with mutations in other genes that contribute to hereditary breast or ovarian cancer such as PALB2, CHEK2, ATM, and Lynch syndrome.

Facing Our Risk of Cancer Empowered (FORCE)

FORCE is a resource for Hereditary Breast and Ovarian Cancer support and advocacy.

www.facingourrisk.org

BRCA Positive Decision Guidance Tool

The BRCA Positive Decision Guidance Tool is an excellent online interactive tool that enables women with BRCA mutations to see what their chances of survival would be after taking different preventative measures at different ages.

http://brcatool.stanford.edu/brca.html

Bright Pink

Bright Pink is an organization specifically for young women who have a BRCA mutation. Its website offers online social networking, support groups, and information about screening and prophylactic surgeries, as well as tips for taking care of oneself following a positive BRCA test result.

www.bebrightpink.org

Breast Reconstruction

For patients considering mastectomy and breast reconstruction, this website offers information about the process and options. It also offers information about insurance coverage, a blog of one woman's experiences, and other resources surrounding this issue.

www.breastrecon.com

His Breast Cancer Awareness

This site and organization provides information about male breast cancer. This page was started by a survivor of male breast cancer, Harvey Singer, together with his wife. Their goal was to provide men with information about breast cancer prevention and treatment.

www.hisbreastcancer.org

John W. Nick Foundation

This organization is dedicated to men with breast cancer.

www.johnwnickfoundation.org

Male Breast Cancer

This is an Australian-based website that is dedicated to men with breast cancer and their families and friends. The website offers up-to-date information regarding male breast cancer facts, treatment options, and life after breast cancer treatment.

http://breastcancerinmen.canceraustralia.gov.au

Men Against Breast Cancer

Men who have a loved one affected with breast cancer can find productive strategies for dealing with their loved one's diagnosis.

www.menagainstbreastcancer.org

National Ovarian Cancer Coalition (NOCC)

The NOCC website offers education and support for individuals concerned about ovarian cancer.

www.ovarian.org

Ovarian Cancer Risk-Reducing Surgery: A Decision-Making Resource

This book is produced by the Margaret Dyson Family Risk Assessment Program and the Fox Chase Cancer Center. Topics include understanding your risk for ovarian cancer, considering risk-reducing surgery, what you need to know if you're having surgery, what you need to know if you decide not to have surgery, and sexuality and intimacy issues. This book is available free of charge by emailing surgerybook@fccc.edu or by viewing a PDF at www.fccc.edu/mobile/ rap-book/Ovarian-Cancer-Risk-Reducing-Surgery.html.

HysterSisters

HysterSisters is a website that offers information about hysterectomies and oophorectomies for both benign and cancerous findings. In addition to information on what to expect before and after surgery, this website offers online support forums, chat rooms, and stories from other women.

www.hystersisters.com

Prophylactic Mastectomy Video Series

Developed by *Glamour* magazine, this video series presents Caitlin Brodnick, a twenty-eight-year-old comedian who tested positive for a BRCA1 gene mutation. Caitlin makes the decision to undergo a preventative double mastectomy. You can follow her on her journey in this documentary series, available in episodes on YouTube.

www.youtube.com/watch?v=czyflOctVQM

Sharsheret

Sharsheret is a national organization of cancer survivors dedicated to addressing the unique concerns of young Jewish women facing breast cancer. Sharsheret has responded to thousands of phone calls from health-care professionals, Jewish organizations, women's organizations, friends and family of women affected by breast cancer, and women affected by breast cancer themselves. Sharsheret's efforts to support young women and educate health-care professionals have been recognized with prestigious awards and significant media coverage.

www.sharsheret.org

Sisters Network Inc.

Sisters Network Inc. is a national African American breast cancer survivorship organization. It provides information and support for African American women with breast cancer and also educates unaffected women. Sisters Network Inc. hosts multiple annual conferences throughout the country in order to reach as many women as possible and it also has financial assistance programs to help pay for mammograms for women who qualify.

www.sistersnetworkinc.org

Susan G. Komen for the Cure

This organization's website has many resources, including information and support for individuals with breast cancer and for their loved ones.

www.komen.org

Young Survival Coalition

The Young Survival Coalition is an organization that is dedicated specifically to issues unique to young women with breast cancer. Their website has lots of information and resources for young women.

www.youngsurvival.org

LI-FRAUMENI SYNDROME (LFS)

Li-Fraumeni Syndrome Association

The LFS Association website provides a wide range of information about advocacy and support services for individuals and families with Li-Fraumeni syndrome. The organization supports a consortium of researchers, medical providers, and caregivers to further research and promote optimal care for the LFS community. It also holds annual conferences around the United States for patients with LFS.

www.lfsassociation.org

Cancer.Net: Li-Fraumeni Syndrome

This website provides an easy-to-understand outline of Li-Fraumeni syndrome. It also has links to Web pages explaining the various types of cancers that can be seen in patients with LFS.

www.cancer.net/cancer-types/li-fraumeni-syndrome

Li-Fraumeni Syndrome Support Group

This is an online community of patients with Li-Fraumeni syndrome.

www.mdjunction.com/li-fraumeni-syndrome

National Institutes of Health: Clinical Trial

A clinical trial funded by the National Institutes of Health. The goals of this study are to learn more about the types of cancers that occur in individuals with LFS, to study the role of the TP53 gene in the development of cancer, to look for other possible genes that cause LFS, to study the effect of LFS diagnoses on families, and to determine if environmental factors or other genes can change a person's cancer risk associated with LFS.

http://clinicalstudies.info.nih.gov/cgi/wais/bold032001 .pl?A_11-C-0255.html@Li-Fraumeni

COWDEN SYNDROME (PTEN MUTATIONS)

PTEN Foundation

The PTEN Foundation was founded to provide hope and financial support to patients, support research, provide education, and promote awareness.

www.ptenfoundation.org

PTEN Previvor Blog

This is an online blog written by a young previvor who was found to have a PTEN mutation. Her story of choosing a double mastectomy to reduce her risk, as well as her day-to-day activities while living with Cowden syndrome, is narrated at this site.

http://tatatothegirls.blogspot.com/2012/10/cowdenssyndrome.html

Pinterest for PTEN Mutations

This is a Pinterest page full of links about Cowden syndrome and PTEN mutations.

www.pinterest.com/emmeili/breast-cancer-and-cowdens-syndrome-85-lifetime-ris

HEREDITARY COLORECTAL CANCER SYNDROMES

Patients with Lynch syndrome, CHEK2 mutations, familial adenomatous polyposis (FAP), and multiple adenomatous polyposis will find these sites useful.

Hereditary Colon Cancer Takes Guts (HCCTG)

HCCTG is a support group for patients to raise awareness about hereditary colon cancer conditions. HCCTG works with other groups to develop patient-friendly resources that can successfully empower families to be strong advocates of their own health care.

www.hcctakesguts.org

Colon Cancer Alliance

This is a website dedicated to individuals with colon cancer or individuals with family or friends with colon cancer. It contains information about living with a colon cancer diagnosis, current clinical trials for colon cancer, treatments for colon cancer, personal stories of survivors, and additional support information.

www.ccalliance.org

Polypeople

This website is a support group for patients and families with FAP and other hereditary polyposis conditions. It provides information about diets, current clinical trials, how to raise awareness about FAP, and ways to contact other individuals with FAP.

www.polypeople.net

FAP Gene

This online support group is based in the United Kingdom and provides informal chat rooms, Facebook links, a newsletter, and other resources for patients with FAP.

www.fapgene.com

PEUTZ-JEGHERS SYNDROME

Peutz-Jeghers Syndrome (PJS) & Juvenile Polyposis Syndrome (JPS) Online Support Group

The PJS & JPS Online Support Group provides information and support for individuals with PJS and JPS, their families, friends, interested medical professionals, and researchers. Patients must sign up via email to join the community and access the various resources.

www.acor.org/listservs/join/114

Smart Patients Peutz-Jeghers Syndrome Community

The Smart Patients Peutz-Jeghers Syndrome community is an online discussion forum where members dealing with PJS, juvenile polyposis syndrome, and familial adenomatous polyposis share advice and support with other patients and caregivers.

www.smartpatients.com/communities/peutz-jeghers -syndrome

HEREDITARY DIFFUSE GASTRIC CANCER (HDGC)

Gastric Cancer Foundation

This is a group that focuses on research, education, and advocacy for patients affected by gastric cancer. This is the first group to form a gastric cancer registry for research but also focus on genetic research.

www.gastriccancer.org

No Stomach for Cancer

No Stomach for Cancer is an international support group with resources regarding gastric cancer and prophylactic gastrectomy. The group also organizes various events to unite patients affected by stomach cancer.

www.nostomachforcancer.org

HEREDITARY KIDNEY CANCER SYNDROMES

Von Hippel–Lindau Syndrome (VHL) Alliance

Von Hippel–Lindau Syndrome Alliance is a family and patient support and research organization for VHL syndrome.

www.vhl.org

Hereditary Leiomyomatosis and Renal Cell Cancer (HLRCC) Family Alliance

HLRCC Family Alliance is a support and research organization for families and patients affected by HLRCC syndrome.

www.hlrccinfo.org

Melanoma Research Foundation (MRF)

The MRF supports medical research to improve melanoma therapy. It educates patients, caregivers, and physicians about the prevention, diagnosis, and treatment of melanoma. The foundation also supports patients with information and forums.

www.melanoma.org

Pancreatic Cancer Action Network

Also useful for patients with PALB2 mutations, the Pancreatic Cancer Action Network is a resource whose primary goals are to advance research, support patients, and create hope for anyone facing pancreatic cancer. It offers online resources and information about clinical trials.

www.pancan.org

GORLIN SYNDROME

Basal Cell Carcinoma Nevus Syndrome (BCCNS) Life Support Network

The BCCNS Life Support Network provides online support and information to individuals with Gorlin syndrome. The group also hosts an annual conference at which individuals can learn the latest information and meet others with the diagnosis.

www.gorlinsyndrome.org

Gorlin Syndrome Group

This is an online website from the United Kingdom. The group offers information about the genetics, surveillance, and treatment for those with Gorlin syndrome.

www.gorlingroup.org

HEREDITARY ENDOCRINE TUMOR PREDISPOSITION SYNDROMES (PARAGANGLIOMA AND PHEOCHROMOCYTOMA AND MEN SYNDROMES)

The Pheo Para Troopers

A Pheo Para Trooper is someone who is passionate about fighting pheochromocytoma and paraganglioma. The goal of this foundation is to empower and support patients while contributing anything they can to finding a cure for these diseases.

www.pheoparatroopers.org

The Pheo Para Alliance

The Pheo Para Alliance is a nonprofit organization with a focus on finding a cure for pheo para through education, research, and fundraising.

www.pheo-para-alliance.org

The Pheochromocytoma Support Board

This is an active online discussion board for patients with pheochromocytomas or paragangliomas.

http://pheochromocytomasupportboard.yuku.com

Association for Multiple Endocrine Neoplasia Disorders (AMEND)

A British website run by patients for patients that informs and supports anyone affected by multiple endocrine neoplasia (MEN) type 1 or 2 or associated endocrine syndromes and tumors. The website offers short videos, discussion forums, information, and more about MEN syndromes and tumors.

www.amend.org.uk

American Multiple Endocrine Neoplasia Support

This website offers seminars, patient connections, and information about MEN syndromes.

www.amensupport.org

The Carcinoid Cancer Foundation

The Carcinoid Cancer Foundation is a nonprofit group for patients with carcinoids and related neuroendocrine tumors. The mission of this foundation is to increase awareness and educate the general public and health-care professionals regarding carcinoid and related neuroendocrine tumors (NETs), to support NET cancer patients and their families, and to serve as patient advocates.

www.carcinoid.org

The National Endocrine and Metabolic Diseases Information Service (NEMDIS)

The NEMDIS website is sponsored by the National Institutes of Health and offers a summary of multiple endocrine neoplasia type 1 (MEN1).

http://endocrine.niddk.nih.gov/pubs/men1/men1.aspx

HEREDITARY PROSTATE CANCER

These are general websites that are not specific to hereditary prostate cancer; the many websites for BRCA mutation carriers are very relevant to hereditary prostate cancer.

Us Too

This group is a prostate cancer education and support group. Us Too provides information about prostate cancer screening, treatments, and new clinical trials.

www.ustoo.org

Prostate Cancer Foundation (PCF)

The PCF website contains comprehensive information about prostate cancer, research opportunities, links for family members and caregivers, and treatment options.

www.pcf.org

NOTES

CHAPTER ONE. KNOWLEDGE THAT CAN SAVE YOUR LIFE

People who carry mutant forms of either of these genes: Sue Friedman, Rebecca Sutphen, and Kathy Steligo, *Confronting Hereditary Breast and Ovarian Cancer* (Baltimore, MD: Johns Hopkins University Press, 2012).

CHAPTER TWO. THE DOUBLE HELIX: BIOLOGY ISN'T DESTINY

"The breasts represent the mothering principle": Louise Hay, *You Can Heal Your Life* (Carlsbad, CA: Hay House, 1984).

It's possible that some sporadic mutations: C. L. Yauk, M. L. Berndt, A. Williams, A. Rowan-Carroll, G. R. Douglas, and M. R. Stämpfli, "Mainstream Tobacco Smoke Causes Paternal Germ-Line DNA Mutation," *Cancer Research* 67, no. 11 (2007): 5103–6; F. Marchetti, A. Rowan-Carroll, A. Williams, A. Polyzos, M. L. Berndt-Weis, and C. L. Yauk, "Sidestream Tobacco Smoke Is a Male Germ Cell Mutagen," *Proceedings of the National Academy of Sciences of the United States of America* 108, no. 31 (2011): 12811–14.

Inherited Cancer Syndromes: National Cancer Institute at the National Institutes of Health, "Genetic Testing for Hereditary Cancer Syndromes," http://www.cancer.gov/cancertopics/fact sheet/Risk/genetic-testing (accessed February 26, 2015).

CHAPTER THREE. TAKING A FAMILY HISTORY: DEALING WITH SILENCE, DEALING WITH DRAMA

A study published by Phuong L. Mai and her colleagues: Phuong L. Mai, Anne O. Garceau, Barry I. Graubard, Marsha Dunn, Timothy S. McNeel, Lou Gonsalves, Mitchell H. Gail, et al., "Confirmation of Cancer Family History Reported in a Population-Based Survey," *Journal of the National Cancer Institute* 103, no. 10 (2011): 788–97.

The Ashkenazi Jewish community provides an example: Dennis Drayna, "Founder Mutations," *Scientific American,* October 2005, 78–85.

The founder effect occurs when a population: N. A. Rosenberg and S. P. Weitzman, "From Generation to Generation: The Genetics of Jewish Populations," *Human Biology: The International Journal of Population Genetics and Anthropology* 85, no. 6 (2013): 817–24.

Ashkenazi ancestry has been traced to about 350 people: S. Carmi, K. Y. Hui, E. Kochav, X. Liu, J. Xue, F. Grady, S. Guha, et al., "Sequencing an Ashkenazi Reference Panel Supports Population-Targeted Personal Genomics and Illuminates Jewish and European Origins," *Nature Communications* 5, no. 4835 (2014).

If you're adopted, here are some ways to get and give important information: Laura Dennis, *Adoption Reunions in the Social Media Age: An Anthology* (Belgrade, Serbia: Entourage Publishing, 2014); Richard Hill, *Finding Family; My Search for Roots and the Secrets in My DNA* (Seattle: CreateSpace Independent Publishing Platform, 2012).

"something that seems like truth—the truth we want to exist": Adam Sternbergh, "Stephen Colbert Has America by the Ballots," *New York Magazine*, October 16, 2006, http://nymag.com /news/politics/22322/index5.html (accessed February 25, 2015).

Studies indicate that a person with a mutation in this gene: A. C. Antoniou, S. Casadei, T. Heikkinen, D. Barrowdale, K. Pylkäs, J. Roberts, A. Lee, et al., "Breast-Cancer Risk in Families with Mutations in PALB2," *New England Journal of Medicine* 371, no. 6 (2014): 497–506.

When the actress Angelina Jolie publicly announced: Angelina Jolie, "My Medical Choice," *New York Times*, May 14, 2013.

CHAPTER SIX. HOW TO MANAGE YOUR CANCER RISK
WHEN INFORMATION IS LIMITED

when you have a family history of endometrial cancer: Michael Blastland and David Spiegelhalter, *The Norm Chronicles: Stories and Numbers about Danger and Death* (New York: Basic Books, 2014).

In 2010, the British medical journal *Lancet* published an essay by Caroline Wellbery: Caroline Wellbery, "The Value of Medical Uncertainty?," *Lancet* 375 (2010): 1686–67.

In a 1995 study published in the *Journal of the American Medical Association*: Donald Redelmeier and Eldar Shafir, "Medical Decision Making in Situations That Offer Multiple Alternatives," *Journal of the American Medical Association* 273 (1995): 302–5.

CHAPTER SEVEN. TARGETED TREATMENTS FOR CANCER:
REALITIES, MYTHS, POSSIBILITIES

The researchers published the family's genetic information in 1998: N. O. Atuk, C. Stolle, J. A. Owen Jr., J. T. Carpenter, and

M. L. Vance, "Pheochromocytoma in Von Hippel–Lindau Disease: Clinical Presentation and Mutation Analysis in a Large, Multigenerational Kindred," *Journal of Clinical Endocrinology and Metabolism* 83 (1998): 117–20.

If they develop advanced kidney cancer: L. Gossage and T. Eisen, "Alterations in VHL as Potential Biomarkers in Renal-Cell Carcinoma," *Nature Reviews Clinical Oncology* 7, no. 5 (2010): 277–88.

"I take my medication and tell everybody something else is going to have to kill me": Jennifer Rainey Marquez, "Together We Stand," *Parade,* August 31, 2014: 9. http://www.epageflip .net/i/373201-august-31-2014/12.

fortunately, there are additional drugs to use when this happens: S. O'Brien, J. P. Radich, C. N. Abboud, M. Ahktari, J. K. Altman, E. Berman, D. J. DeAngelo, et al., "Chronic Myelogenous Leukemia, Version 1.2014," *Journal of the National Comprehensive Cancer Network* 11, no. 11 (2013): 1327–40.

Only *half* the breast cancer patients who start on tamoxifen: C. Davies, J. Godwin, R. Gray, et al., "Relevance of Breast Cancer Hormone Receptors and Other Factors to the Efficacy of Adjuvant Tamoxifen: Patient-Level Meta-Analysis of Randomised Trials," *Lancet* 378, no. 9793 (2011): 771–84; C. A. Sawka, K. I. Pritchard, W. Shelley, G. DeBoer, A. H. Paterson, J. W. Meakin, and D. J. Sutherland, "A Randomized Crossover Trial of Tamoxifen versus Ovarian Ablation for Metastatic Breast Cancer in Premenopausal Women: A Report of the National Cancer Institute of Canada Clinical Trials Group (NCIC CTG) Trial MA.1," *Breast Cancer Research and Treatment* 44, no. 3 (1997): 211–15.

tamoxifen reduces risk in high-risk patients: Victor G. Vogel, Joseph P. Constantino, D. Lawrence Wickerham, Walter M. Cronin, Reena S. Ceccini, James N. Atkins, Terese B. Bevers, Louis Fehrenbacher, et al., "Update of the NSABP STAR P-2

Trial: Preventing Breast Cancer," *Cancer Prevention Research* 3, no. 7 (2010): 696–706.

It works on tumors that make a mutated form of a kinase: Thomas J. Lynch, Daphne W. Bell, Raffaella Sordella, Sarada Gurubhagavatula, Ross A. Okimoto, Brian W. Brannigan, Patricia L. Harris, et al., "Activating Mutations in the Epidermal Growth Factor Receptor Underlying Responsiveness of Non–Small-Cell Lung Cancer to Gefitinib," *New England Journal of Medicine* 350 (2004): 2129–39; J. Guillermo Paez, Pasi A. Jänne, Jeffrey C. Lee, Sean Tracy, Heidi Greulich, Stacey Gabriel, Paula Herman, et al., "EGFR Mutations in Lung Cancer: Correlation with Clinical Response to Gefitinib Therapy," *Science* 204 (2004): 1497–500.

Vandetanib targets the VEGF receptor and other kinases: E. N. Imyanitov and T. Byrski, "Systemic Treatment for Hereditary Cancers: A 2012 Update," *Hereditary Cancer in Clinical Practice* 11, no. 1 (2013): 2.

in cultured cells, iniparib did not appear to be a standard PARP inhibitor after all: G. Patel, S. B. DeLorenzo, K. S. Flatten, G. G. Poirier, and S. H. Kaufmann, "Failure of Iniparib to Inhibit Poly(ADP-Ribose) Polymerase in Vitro," *Clinical Cancer Research* 18, no. 6 (2012): 1655–62; X. Liu, Y. Shi, D. X. Maag, J. P. Palma, M. J. Patterson, P. A. Ellis, B. W. Surber, et al., "Iniparib Nonselectively Modifies Cysteine-Containing Proteins in Tumor Cells and Is Not a Bona Fide PARP Inhibitor," *Clinical Cancer Research* 18, no. 2 (2012): 510–23.

iniparib could still be a successful drug: Joyce O'Shaughnessy, Lee Schwartzberg, Michael A. Danso, et al., "Phase III Study of Iniparib plus Gemcitabine and Carboplatin versus Gemcitabine and Carboplatin in Patients with Metastatic Triple-Negative Breast Cancer," *Journal of Clinical Oncology* 32, no. 34 (2014): 3840–47.

PARP inhibition can delay the development of breast cancers in mice with BRCA1 mutations: Ciric To, Eun-Hee Kim, Darlene B. Royce, Charlotte R. Williams, Ryan M. Collins, Renee Risingsong, Michael B. Sporn, and Karen T. Liby, "The PARP Inhibitors, Veliparib and Olaparib, Are Effective Chemopreventive Agents for Delaying Mammary Tumor Development in BRCA1-Deficient Mice," *Cancer Prevention Research,* http://cancerpreventionresearch.aacrjournals.org/content/early/2014/05/09/1940-6207.CAPR-14-0047 (accessed February 26, 2015).

its entry into the clinic has significantly improved the prognosis for HER2 positive breast cancers: Edith A. Perez, Edward H. Romond, Vera J. Suman, Jong Hyeon Jeong, George Sledge, Charles E. Geyer Jr., Silvana Martino, et al., "Trastuzumab Plus Adjuvant Chemotherapy for Human Epidermal Growth Factor Receptor 2–Positive Breast Cancer: Planned Joint Analysis of Overall Survival from NSABP B-31 and NCCTG N9831," *Journal of Clinical Oncology* 32 (2014): 3744.

twenty-seven of thirty patients had a complete remission after treatment with CAR T cells: Shannon L. Maude, Noelle Frey, Pamela A. Shaw, Richard Aplenc, David M. Barrett, Nancy J. Bunin, Anne Chew, et al., "Chimeric Antigen Receptor T Cells for Sustained Remissions in Leukemia," *New England Journal of Medicine* 371 (2014): 1507–17.

ipilimumab and nivolumab are indeed synergistic: Michael A. Postow, Jason Chesney, Anna C. Pavlick, Caroline Robert, Kenneth Grossmann, David McDermott, Gerald P. Linette, et al., "Nivolumab and Ipilimumab versus Ipilimumab in Untreated Melanoma," *New England Journal of Medicine* 372, no. 21 (2015): 2006–17.

side effects do limit their use: Mark Fuerst, "Separating the Hope, Hype, and Reality of Precision Medicine," *Oncology Times* 37, no. 3 (2015): 1, 16–18.

researchers compared results of the surgery to a sham version of the operation: R. Sihvonen, M. Paavola, A. Malmivaara, A. Itälä, A. Joukainen, H. Nurmi, J. Kalske, T. L. Järvinen, and Finnish Degenerative Meniscal Lesion Study (FIDELTY) Group, "Arthroscopic Partial Meniscectomy versus Sham Surgery for a Degenerative Meniscal Tear," *New England Journal of Medicine* 369, no. 26 (2013): 2515–24.

the BRAF gene was discovered to be mutated in more than 50 percent of melanomas: H. Davies, G. R. Bignell, C. Cox, P. Stephens, S. Edkins, S. Clegg, and J. Teague, "Mutations of the BRAF Gene in Human Cancer," *Nature* 417, no. 6892 (2012): 949–54.

Vemurafenib and its cousins work only in patients whose tumors have the BFAF V600E mutation: K. T. Flaherty, I. Pazanov, K. B. Kim, A. Ribas, G. A. McArthur, J. A. Sosman, P. J. O'Dwyer, et al., "Inhibition of Mutated, Activated BRAF in Metastatic Melanoma," *New England Journal of Medicine* 363, no. 9 (2010): 809–19.

BRAF-mutant colon cancers insensitive to BRAF inhibitors: A. Prahallad, C. Sun, S. Huang, F. Di Nicolantonio, R. Salazar, D. Zecchin, R. L. Beijersbergen, A. Bardelli, and R. Bernards, "Unresponsiveness of Colon Cancer to BRAF (V600E) Inhibition through Feedback Activation of EGFR," *Nature* 483, no. 7387 (2012): 100–3; R. B. Corcoran, H. Ebi, A. B. Turke, E. M. Coffee, M. Nishino, A. P. Cogdill, R. D. Brown, et al., "EGFR-Mediated Re-Activation of MAPK Signaling Contributes to Insensitivity of BRAF Mutant Colorectal Cancers to RAF Inhibition with Vemurafenib," *Cancer Discovery* 3, no. 2 (2012): 227–35; M. Mao, F. Tian, J. M. Mariadason, C. C. Tsao, R. Lemos Jr., F. Dayyani, Y. N. Gopal, et al., "Resistance to BRAF Inhibition in BRAF-Mutant Colon Cancer Can Be Overcome with P13K Inhibition or Demethylating Agents," *Clinical Cancer Research* 19, no. 3 (2013): 657–67.

lawsuits against insurance companies that refused to pay for bone marrow transplants: Erik Eckholm, "$89 Million Awarded Family Who Sued H.M.O.," *New York Times,* December 30, 1993.

insurance companies were increasing their premiums: H. Gilbert Welch and Juliana Mogielnicki, "Presumed Benefit: Lesson from the American Experience with Marrow Transplantation for Breast Cancer," *British Medical Journal* 324, no. 7345 (2002): 1088–92.

Come to our cancer treatment center: S. W. Gray, A. Cronin, E. Bair, N. Lindeman, V. Viswanath, and K. A. Janeway, "Marketing of Personalized Cancer Care on the Web: An Analysis of Internet Websites," *Journal of the National Cancer Institute* 107, no. 5 (2015): djv030.

CHAPTER EIGHT. SCIENCE IS A GROUP PROJECT: DATA POINTS AND YOU

As an article in *Science Translational Medicine* in 2011 concluded: Callum J. Bell, Darrell L. Dinwiddie, Neil A. Miller, Shannon L. Hateley, Elena E. Ganusova, Joanna Mudge, Ray J. Langley, et al., "Carrier Testing for Severe Childhood Recessive Diseases by Next-Generation Sequencing," *Science Translational Medicine* 3, no. 65 (2011): 65ra4 or 1–14.

Too much is made of research on very small numbers of people: D. G. MacArthur, T. A. Manolio, D. P. Dimmock, H. L. Rehm, J. Shendure, G. R. Abecasis, and D. R. Adams, "Guidelines for Investigating Causality in Sequence Variants in Human Disease," *Nature* 508 (2014): 469–76.

first cancer cell line to grow indefinitely in a culture dish: Rebecca Skloot, *The Immortal Life of Henrietta Lacks* (New York: Broadway Books, 2011).

In 2013, a controversy erupted: Melissa Gymrek, Amy L. McGuire, David Golan, Erin Halperin, and Yaniv Erlich, "Identifying Personal Genomes by Surname Inference," *Science* 339, no. 6117 (2013): 321–24.

there are also policy, legal, and information technology hurdles: Francis S. Collins and Margaret A. Hamburg, "First FDA Authorization for Next-Generation Sequencer," *New England Journal of Medicine* 369 (2013): 2369–71.

My own lab just reported on our analyses of the sequences of the whole genomes: Samantha B. Foley, Jonathan J. Rios, Victoria E. Mgbemena, Linda S. Robinson, Heather L. Hampel, Amanda E. Toland, Leslie Durham, and Theodora S. Ross, "Use of Whole Genome Sequencing for Diagnosis and Discovery in the Cancer Genetics Clinic," *EbioMedicine* 2, no. 1 (2014): 74–81.

mutations in BRCA1: D. E. Goldgar, L. A. Cannon-Albright, A. Oliphant, J. H. Ward, G. Linker, J. Swensen, T. D. Tran, et al., "Chromosome 17q Linkage Studies of 18 Utah Breast Cancer Kindreds," *American Journal of Human Genetics* 52 (1993): 743–48.

BRCA2: V. Tavtigian, J. Simard, J. Rommens, F. Couch, D. Shattuck-Eidens, S. Neuhausen, S. Merajver, et al., "The Complete BRCA2 Gene and Mutations in Chromosome 13q-Linked Kindreds," *Nature Genetics* 12, no. 3 (1996): 333–37.

APC (the familial adenomatous polyposis colon cancer gene): L. N. Spirio, W. Samowitz, J. Robertson, M. Robertson, R. W. Burt, M. Leppert, and R. White, "Alleles of APC Modulate the Frequency and Classes of Mutations That Lead to Colon Polyps," *Nature Genetics* 20, no. 4 (1998): 385–88; Y. Nakamura, I. Nishisho, K. W. Kinsler, B. Vogelstein, Y. Miyoshi, Y. Miki, H. Ando, A. Horri, et al., "Mutations of the APC (Adenomatous Polyposis Coli) Gene in FAP (Familial Polyposis Coli) Patients and in Sporadic Colorectal Tumors," *Journal of Experimental Medicine* 168, no. 2 (1992): 141–47.

CDKN2A (known as the "melanoma gene"): A. Kamb, D. Shattuck-Eidens, R. Eiles, Q. Liu, N. A. Gruis, W. Ding, C. Hussey, T. Tran, Y. Miki, et al., "Analysis of the p16 Gene (CDKN2) as a Candidate for Chromosome 9p Melanoma Susceptibility Locus," *Nature Genetics* 8, no. 1 (1994): 22–26.

INDEX

RB1 gene, 215–16
Redelmeier, Donald, 141
reference genome, 104
relationships, genogram and, 46–47, 49
renal cancer
    CHEK2 gene and, 203
    FH gene and, 210
    FLCN gene and, 210–11
    Lynch syndrome and, 207–8
    MITF gene and, 212
    PTEN gene and, 204–5, 213–14
    sarcomas, 215
research. *See* clinical research
research number, 186
resistance, 156
resources, 253–66
RET gene, 28, 88, 129, 158, 214–15
retinoblastoma, 215–16
reunions, collecting family medical
    data at, 54
rhabdoid tumor predisposition, 219
Right Action for Women (the "Applegate
    Fund"), 101
risks and risk management
    complexity of, 142
    expressed in percentages, 79–80
    managing, 8, 121–46
    process of, 124–26
    range of, 106
Robinson, Linda, 99
"the Rocket" (BRCA2 mutation cancer
    patient), 77–78
Rosenberg, Noah, 60
Rosenblum, Jacob. *See* Jack (author's uncle)
Ross, Theodora (author)
    BRCA1 gene and, xiv, 59, 72, 98–100,
        107–8, 116
    BRCA2 gene and, 98, 99
    childhood of, 39–43, 139
    genetic counseling and, 4, 6, 94–95, 98–100,
        102, 116
    genetic testing and, 1–2, 99, 107–8
    informing family about tests, 116–20
    medical records of, 81–82
    melanoma of, 2, 59, 92–93, 108, 132
    notifying coworkers and friends, 132–33
    privacy and, 132–33
    prophylactic surgeries of, 7, 126–27,
        132, 140
    reactions of, 6–7, 73–74, 140, 144
    reconstructive surgery of, 136–37, 143
    reduced cancer risk of, 195–96
    training and career of, xiv, 2–3, 18–19,
        59, 131

Ross/Rosenblum family
    BRCA genes and, 59–62, 67, 107–8,
        116–17, 184–86
    cancers in, 30–35
    CBP gene and, 183, 186
    genetic testing and, 107–8, 116–20, 196
    research study and, 31, 63, 72,
        180–86, 195
    secrecy in, 32–34, 39, 45–46
    See also names of family members
RPS19 gene, 221
Rubinstein-Taybi syndrome, 183

Sanger sequencing, 103
Sanofi (drug company), 160–61
SBDS gene, 220
schwannomas, 218–19
Science, 188
Science Translational Medicine, 183–84
scientific method, 172
screenings, 125, 136
SDH genes, 213–14
Sean (author's husband)
    analysis by, 73, 140
    genetic testing and, 2–3, 4, 59
    helping with family research, 64
second opinions, 81, 135
secrecy
    in author's family, 32–33, 39, 45–46
    about ethnic heritage, 65–66
    medical history and, 11–12, 43–44
self-deception, 87
sequencer, 103
Sertoli cell tumors, 218–19
Shafir, Eldar, 141
SHAF2 gene, 213–14
Shwachman-Diamond syndrome, 220
side effects
    of tamoxifen, 155
    targeted therapies and, 150–51,
        167–68
Siegel, Bernie, 17, 18
single-strand breaks in DNA, 160
skin cancer, 202, 207–8, 220
Skolnick, Mark, 194
SLX4 gene, 216
SMAD4 gene, 209
small intestine cancer, 28, 206, 207–8, 208–9
small-molecule kinase inhibitors, 157, 162
SMARCB1 gene, 219
smoking, 23
social media, 54
soft-tissue sarcoma, 27, 202, 215
solid tumors, 221